Turning Point

Discovering the Simple Secrets to
Health, Happiness, and Wholeness

by Wilson Adams

Foreword by Professional Fitness Trainer
Carter Hays

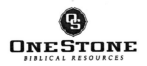

ONESTONE
BIBLICAL RESOURCES

© 2013 One Stone Press – All rights reserved.

No part of this publication may be reproduced, stored in a retrieval system, or transmitted in any way by any means—electronic, mechanical, photocopy, recording, or otherwise—without the prior permission of the copyright holder, except as provided by USA copyright law.

Scripture references marked NIV are taken from the *Holy Bible, New International Version*®. NIV®. Copyright © 1973, 1978, 1984 by the International Bible Society. Used by permission of Zondervan. All rights reserved.

Scripture references marked NASB are taken from the *New American Standard Bible*®, © 1960, 1962, 1963, 1968, 1971, 1972, 1973, 1975, 1977, 1995 by The Lockman Foundation. Used by permission. (www.Lockman.org)

Scripture references marked NKJV are taken from the *New King James Version*. Copyright © 1982 by Thomas Nelson, Inc. Used by permission. All rights reserved.

Contents

Acknowledgments

A book is never the project of one, but it requires the quintessential team effort. I am indebted to all those who contributed to this message. A special thanks to Carter Hays for his willingness to write the Foreword. He is one of the busiest people I know, often beginning his day while the rest of the world sleeps. It was hearing him speak early on that provided the spark that ignited these thoughts. To four people willing to share their struggles and stories—Andrew, Kate, Michelle, and Tracy—I count each of you as friends. To all those who consented to interviews and who sent responses to my questions that eventually found their way into the book, thank you. Your insight in areas of expertise added much. To Andy, Joy, Greg, April, and the team at One Stone in Bowling Green, Kentucky who encouraged the project and saw it through, this could have not been accomplished without you.

To my wife Julie, I offer a very special word of thanks. She turned the corner with me and was willing to share her story. It wasn't easy, but she did it in the hopes that it would help others in their struggle. She read the manuscript, made helpful suggestions and corrections, and kept encouraging me through the process. I could not have done it without her.

To my dad and stepmother whose examples prove that a common sense approach of moderation and exercise really works—thanks for staying engaged and staying young. You inspire all of us! To Luke, our last of four children and the only one left at home while Dad wrote this book—I promise I won't stand behind you any more at a restaurant and tell you how many grams of sodium are in the sandwich you just ordered

Foremost, I offer a very special word of appreciation to you, the reader. I hope something within these pages will cause you to pause, perhaps smile, but most of all, take inventory. Each of us has been given the gift of life. And since you don't get a do-over, you better make this one count. And if you need the impetus for your own *Turning Point*, I hope you find it. Thanks for reading and sharing your time. It is valued.

Foreword

I have been blessed throughout my lifetime to help people create optimal health and peak performance. During the last 12 years a significant amount of my time has been spent helping people in their struggle with the insidious effects of obesity.

I have always viewed physical training; be it for athletics, fitness, or physical problems, as a gift from the Lord to help others. Through my wellness work I have met hundreds of caring and compassionate people with a similar passion. Sharing the Gospel was never meant to be limited to the "door to door" approach familiar to so many. I feel compelled to share the message of love, hope, and faith in Christ through the creation of a vibrant healthy lifestyle.

It was through one of my wellness talks that I was honored to meet Wilson Adams. I was at an event speaking on spiritual wellness and the necessity of supporting a healthy diet with Juice Plus+. Being like-minded with the passion to help others thrive towards their God-given potential we became good friends. I was blessed to be able to train Julie, Wilson's wife, and help support her journey to forge a lifestyle of health, and fitness.

There are literally thousands of books on health, fitness, wellness, diet, exercise, and whatever your need for whatever is! In *Turning Point* you will find simple, faith-based solutions to the health challenges so many people are facing today. You are going to find solace in the following pages as Wilson weaves the stories, testimonies, anecdotes, and winning strategies of "real people" becoming the masters of their decisions rather than mastered by their circumstances.

Relevance is based on shared experience. We are a nation that is pummeled daily with a morass of misinformation on health and fitness. Wilson cuts expertly through the rhetoric and statistics, and delivers faith-driven common sense. Truth is only found through the Word of God. Therefore faith must be present with common sense health strategies or you can become susceptible to the hype and not the hope.

You and I live in the real world. We are bombarded with food choices, narratives on food choices, and crazy diets that on their best day make no sense. We are encouraged to do this exercise routine, get that DVD, go high intensity exercise, or go slow and steady, UGH! Relax, you have found safe refuge in *Turning Point*. Wilson gives you fundamental truths on diet, living an active lifestyle, along with safe and effective exercise. The testimonies you are going to read represent where you've been, where you are, or where you are going to be. The truth is this; where you are now, is not who you are. As you read the stories you are going to hear where these people were in their life, but they discovered that is NOT who they are. I encourage you to read Psalm 139 to hear who God created you to be. You my friend are ... "fearfully and wonderfully made."

As you read *Turning Point* I encourage you to frame Wilson's message through the motto: *I Can. I Am. I Do.*

I Can

God does not download "I cannot" into our human software. God is the creator of your unlimited potential, the giver of your unique gifts and talents. You have been placed here at this time for a specific purpose. I believe you are the only one who can fulfill that purpose in the way God intended it to be carried forth.

My humble suggestion is to first get to know your Creator, personally. **God's will for you is found in His Word.** Read Scripture to get to know your Father. In doing so you will learn what He wants you to do. Remember: the only difference between *can* and *cannot* is the **NOT**. Drop it. It's not the right voice to hear.

I Am

I AM was the name of God given to Moses on the mountain when He asked; "Who should I say sent me?" I AM literally translates to, "I am *that* which you need." What strikes me about this declaration ["I am that which you need"] is that it isn't so much about our past or future as it is about the now—this moment. The more we can live our lives in this moment, the less apt we are to live in the mindset of past troubles or future problems. This is how we start, work through, and achieve goals in our life.

I recommend the *I Am* process. "*I am* in the process of (your goal) by (specific date). For example; "*I am* in the process of losing 50 pounds by December 1." We are all in the process of becoming. The more we can laser focus through *I Am* thinking, the better we are able to avoid the *I Will*. *I Will* is tomorrow and tomorrow never tends to happen. Tomorrow is the seed of the most virulent virus ever created, procrastination. Procrastination is a disease of the soul that will rob you of the joy of accomplishment. Procrastination is code-named "excuses." "Today's excuses are tomorrow's failures." They are the seeds of shame, guilt, and remorse. They are weeds. You till the soil of success and victory through *I Am*, then the seeds you plant today will always bear the fruit of passion, joy, humility, and achievement.

I Do

I Do brings full circle the *I Am* and *I Can*. If we have the power of *I Am* with no follow through, we can never fully believe in the *I Can*, and ultimately know "Who we are." The challenge for all of us is in the *I Do*. *I Do* is the committed follow through that belief and faith must fuel. The battle of our journey is typically in the *I Do* arena. That's where we deal with things emotionally, and it is in the emotions we are most susceptible to the lie of *I Cannot*. Remember that every area of your life is weaved with hope. If you don't have hope, you have bought the lie.

Living by Intention

To live with intention is a powerful theme throughout this book. It dramatically affects our spiritual, mental, and most certainly our physical life. God created everything He desired through His Word; He spoke it into existence. By harnessing our thoughts with His Word, declaring out loud our intentions, and then acting upon them, we follow the pattern He Himself created.

Throughout this book you are given opportunities to challenge your way of thinking, to discover your divine destiny through God's Word. When you have your thoughts in alignment with God's plan for you, then you are positioned to speak life into your lifestyle. Speaking words of faith sprout from belief, and to believe with your whole heart is sown from trusting God.

To lose weight, to become fit, to be all that the Lord created you to be is revealed in the stories and fundamental strategies for health in the following pages. For example, when you meet Andrew you'll meet a kind, gentle, and compassionate man. Andrew was well over 400 pounds when I met him and all I could see was his potential. We first must learn to see with our heart before our eyes.

I am writing this forward because I believe in Wilson Adams' love and deep commitment to help others. I believe we are all given incredible gifts so that we might give back. I look forward to reading your personal story someday because this book helped you take the first step to unleash your unlimited potential. We always take the first step seemingly alone, yet we soon discover the Lord is our #1 cheerleader.

—Carter Hays; CES, PES, FSN
Author—*Discover Your Road to Divine Health*
Franklin, Tennessee

Note to the Reader

This book is about life. It's about challenging you to live your days to their fullest while maximizing your health, vitality, and availability for God. The Creator and Savior deserve more than our leftovers—He deserves our very best. After all, you only get one life, so make the most of it. "As for the days of our life, they contain seventy years, or if due to strength, eighty years... So teach us to number our days, that we may present to You a heart of wisdom" (Psalm 90:10, 12). Paul said it this way: "Make the most of every opportunity..." (Ephesians 5:16).

I am amazed at the approaches people take to this subject. First, most go around it and refuse to touch it. Second, we tend to go to extremes—either throw-caution-to-the-wind on one hand ("see no evil, hear no evil, taste no evil") or portray know-it-all neurosis on the other. Third, most books on the subject leave out the most important element is the equation: the spiritual side of man. Jesus connected the spiritual to the physical when He said, "Man shall not live on bread alone, but on every word that proceeds from the mouth of God" (Matt.4:4). Because man is a dual being, to discuss this subject without acknowledging the critical *spiritual* component is to miss the motivation as to *why* we should take care of our physical selves.

Regardless, it is a highly charged and polarizing subject. I get that. I only ask for one thing: a fair hearing. I have tried to be biblical while simultaneously urging a common-sense approach. I hope something within these pages will spur your own thinking and motivate you to make whatever life improvements you need to make.

I recently visited a friend my age. He has become almost completely sedentary. He is struggling with severe health issues (diabetes and heart). He didn't get that way overnight and he won't be fixed overnight—if at all. I'm very concerned about him. By his own admission, he hasn't always made good choices. One thing led to another, until he is in the shape he's in today. Sadly, he is one in a multitude.

Anyone who would dare write about this will open himself up to criticism. I've learned over time, however, that critics seldom evaluate fairly (they may not even read the book) and/or jump to conclusions that are unwarranted. That will be true especially on this extremely touchy subject.

Obviously no book replaces the diagnostic expertise and medical advice of a licensed professional. It is essential that you consult your doctor before making any decisions involving physical exercise or changes in diet that could affect your health. I am not a medical doctor, psychologist, psychotherapist, psychiatrist, personal trainer, nutritionist, etc., and thus not qualified to give health, exercise, diet, or medical-related advice. And ditto for my publisher. If you stand in need of help in any of those areas, consult a qualified professional.

What I am is this: an observant disciple of life who is willing to share some insight about what he has learned along the bumps and bruises of the journey. I can read, study, research, observe, interview, etc., and pass along an accumulation of information. At the end of the day, however, you are the guardian of your life and the choices you make are yours to make. And that is the basic premise of this book.

Neither do my references to the NBC program, *The Biggest Loser*, imply that I endorse everything about the popular television reality show. It is, after all, *television*—which includes elements of drama and entertainment. As a result, the values and opinions offered on the BL program by all parties do not necessarily reflect the author's views or that of my publisher.

The same principle applies to those interviewed and referenced in this book. An endorsement of one's opinion on a subject wherein he/she is qualified to speak does not necessarily reflect the author's endorsement of everything they believe or have ever said (and vice versa).

I have no interest in writing a book like a college thesis paper or a doctorial dissertation. As a result, you won't find these pages filled with endless footnotes. A source is cited when deemed appropriate and necessary. I read a statistic recently claiming that "50% of all statistics are made up." That's striking, but only if that statistic is true. I assure the reader that I have no interest in fabrication to sensationalize a story. Truth, after all, is stranger (and scarier!) than fiction. Those interested in further documentation can find it easily via Internet search engines which can lead you to detailed information on any number of academic and clinical studies related to this subject.

—Wilson Adams
Murfreesboro, Tennessee

To Connie and Bobby Adams—
my dad and step-mother.
You have touched and changed the lives of many.
You mean the world to me.

Introduction

John Maxwell knows his stuff and his stuff is...*leadership*. His books on the subject have sold more than eighteen million copies. John told me a couple years ago that everything he has learned about leadership, he learned from...*the Bible*. Surprised? John Maxwell doesn't force his faith on anyone and neither do I. That said; here's a second secret to share: the fundamental basics of what *I* have learned about health, happiness, and wholeness is *rooted* (pun intended) in...*the Bible*. For that, I make no apology.

You don't have to read very far in the first book of Scripture to learn that in the beginning God created man and placed him in a *garden*. He then gave this simple instruction:

> Behold, I have given you every plant yielding seed that is on the surface of the earth, And every tree which has fruit yielding seed; it shall be food for you. (Genesis 1:29)

And while God later approved the eating of meat (Genesis 9:3), Scripture advocates moderation rather than gluttony. The wise man said, "Put a knife to your throat if you are a man of great appetite" (Proverbs 23:2). Whoa! Apparently the Creator takes this eating thing seriously.

We are what we eat! Certainly no one in the age of instant access and information can take issue with that. The problem, however, isn't information, but motivation. We know yet choose to look the other way. However, the days of rejoicing in blissful ignorance are over. It's time we had a serious discussion and face the facts of twenty-first century reality.

Food addiction (the untouchable subject) has become public health crisis number one.

Here is a sampling of the sad reality of our times:

- 1 in 3 Americans have cardiovascular disease (Center for Disease Control—CDC)

- 2 out of 3 Americans are overweight or obese (CDC)

- 12.5 million children (ages 2 to 19) are obese—three times as many as in the 1980s.(*Journal of the American Medical Association*)

- 1 in 3 women and 1 in 2 men will develop cancer (National Cancer Institute)

- By 2050, 1 in 3 adults (and children) will develop diabetes (CDC)

- More than 25% of American children are on prescription drugs (*Wall Street Journal*)

- By age 12, many of our children have developed the beginning stages of hardening of the arteries (Bogalusa Heart Study)

- A stunning 80% of U.S. teenagers are eating diets that put them on a clear path to heart disease (NBC News)

- U.S. healthcare expenditures are approaching 3 trillion dollars per year (Center for Medicare/Medicaid Services—www.CMS.gov)

If over half of American adults are overweight and one quarter of the population clinically obese (defined as a body mass index of 30 or above), you would think we would wake up (especially given the shocking statistic that obesity rates among our children have more than doubled since 1980). It is estimated that by 2030, 42% of Americans can expect to be obese. Mika Brezezinski reports in her book, *Obsessed*, that four former members of the president's cabinet—two secretaries of agriculture and two secretaries of health and human services—issued a report calling obesity "the most urgent public health problem in America today."

If you think none of this affects you, think again. The same report blamed escalating health-care costs on obesity-related illnesses. Diabetes, the biggest elephant in the health-care crisis room, is linked to obesity. Doctors are becoming alarmed as they see the early signs of this debilitating disease in younger children. Heart disease is also linked to obesity as is joint replacement surgery. Any honest orthopedic surgeon will admit that many of his surgeries are a direct result of overweight patients. Scientists at the Mayo Clinic say the extra medical costs associated with obese patients are even greater than the health costs associated with smoking (*Journal of Occupational and Environmental Medicine*, March 2012). In other words... Ka-ching. Ka-ching. And who pays? You do.

Sugar, salt, and fat has so shaped our diets that these staples of the food industry have shaped us. Would you be surprised to learn that the number one reason for disqualification for military service is...*overweight?* Army generals have testified on Capitol Hill that America's kids are getting "too fat to fight."

Even though we are the sickest people on the planet, we continue to whistle past the all-you-can-eat-buffet-bar while pretending everything is fine. But everything isn't fine. And even though we are living longer, we're not living better or healthier. Health and Fitness Trainer Carter Hays writes, "On the surface you would think everyone would have a passion for a healthy lifestyle, right? More often than not many people have a *wish* not to be unhealthy. There is a monumental difference in these two viewpoints. It really boils down to this: Are you delaying your death, or LIVING your life?"

It's more than a great question. It's a life-changing question. Dr. David Katz, M.D. (Founding Director of Yale University Prevention Research Center and Editor of *Childhood Obesity Journal*) said, "This may be the first generation of children to have a shorter life-span than their parents." Stop and read that again. Does it get your attention? It should. We are eating ourselves to disease and death and allowing our children to do the same.

Your body is a temple... That's biblical (1 Corinthians 6:19-20). We are quick to teach teens about the dangers of drinking, drugs, smoking, etc., with the understanding that we are stewards over our bodies. Is it too much of a stretch to make the same application to food addiction? It's time we had a discussion on this subject the same as we talk about smoking or any other addictive behavior. "You, therefore, who teach another, do you not teach yourself?" (Romans 2:21). It's a serious question.

For the record and before we even get started, I am not a vegetarian (neither am I the food police, food Nazi, etc.). We've all been out to eat with a family member or friend and seen eyes roll when he/she makes a big deal over the menu and announces pompously to everyone present, "My—diet—won't—allow—me—to—eat—*that...*" Great. Pack your bags because we're all going on *their* guilt trip...

I have no desire to be seen as radical or extreme. In fact, taking the *all things in moderation* approach means that you don't have to be extreme. I like a good hamburger as much as the next guy. And an occasional bowl of ice-cream won't kill you (my favorite is any flavor under the Texas label of Blue Bell). So, don't lump me with radical extremism. However, since we broached the subject of radical, I'll say this: having a surgeon open the chest of a forty-year-old for a heart by-pass *is* radical. And diabetes *is* radical. And chemotherapy *is* radical. And so are other chronic health issues we face in record and disturbing numbers. And while some illnesses are equally hereditary as they are dietary, the medical research doesn't lie. Pediatrician and author Dr. Bill Sears declared, "75% of all chronic disease is preventable." Are you kidding? No.

Have we become gluttons for punishment? Walk into a favored fast-food restaurant and the first question asked—"Do you want it SUPER-SIZED?" *Really?* Americans have become infatuated (careful with that word) with "the more the merrier" food portions and happily indulge with a wink and a nod. Given the statistics, it's not funny any more.

In the course of this book I want to get two things into your head.

First, the fix is in...*your head*. The decision to live wiser and better takes place in your mind long before it reaches your fork. "For as he thinks within himself, so is he" (Proverbs 23:7a). Win the battle of the mind and the body will follow. And while it is impossible to stop the effects of physical aging as the body begins its demise, you can slow down the process so you can not only live longer, but live better. But first, you must discipline your thinking. How badly do you want to change? Talk is cheap. Words are easy. Action and positive results, however, takes work.

Second, you must make the decision to become *proactive* about your health. No one will do it for you—not the government, not the food corporate giants, not the restaurants, not the supermarkets—only *you* have control over your daily disciplines. And good intentions are…well, good *intentions*. At the end of the day they accomplish zero, nada, nothing. You must get off the couch or out of the Lazy Boy (an odd and apt description for many of us) and start eating better, drinking more water, and exercising more frequently. Excuses do not work anymore. Fictional fitness doesn't work any more. Only functional fitness delivers.

Sadly, pharmaceutical companies have conditioned us to respond to health-care issues *after the fact*. It never dawns on us that drug companies make much of their money treating the symptoms of illnesses, many of which we bring upon ourselves. And they make a lot of money doing so. And so do some lawyers. It's why daytime television is full of two things: (1) pharmaceutical ads that all end with the same admonition—"Ask your doctor if _____ is right for you," and (2) lawyer ads that implore you to sue the pharmaceutical companies for the side affects of their drugs. It would be funny if it weren't so serious.

There is another cultural enigma that goes unnoticed. Across America there are two businesses on most city street corners: fast-food restaurants offering cheap processed fatty foods and drug stores selling medicines to offset illnesses caused by the cheap processed fatty foods. Few are those who connect the dots. (There is actually another business occupying street corners: gas stations that sell fuel for our cars along with quick/convenient overpriced junk food/fuel for our bodies). And while we know that much of the fast-food offerings are not good for us, we indulge anyway because quick and convenient has become the mantra of the American lifestyle. Eventually, however, too many food stops at the burger joint or the gas-and-go will ultimately lead up the path to the pharmacy on the opposite corner—where they gladly display the welcome mat. And the cycle continues.

Let's be frank (even though my name isn't Frank). Doctors and medicines are often an essential part of maintaining good health. My purpose is not to deride them in any way. I have friends in both fields and will use some of their testimonies in this book. In fact, God has allowed man to gain life-saving and life-prolonging insight in the field of medicine—for which we should all be grateful.

However, there is only so much that physicians and pharmacies can do to treat symptoms that have accumulated over a lifetime of bad choices. And while we shake our head at the nicotine addict who continues to smoke in spite of needing oxygen (because his lungs are all but destroyed by his habit), we can easily be guilty of the *same thing* when it comes to our food choices. We eat too much junk and do so knowing it will eventually catch up to us.

Look around. I see more and more people in my peer group (the middle-age 50s) facing serious health-related issues because of bad lifestyle habits they developed in their earlier years. It *has* caught up to them. Some may even be past the point of no return. That's sad. Not only is it tragic for them personally, but also for their families. It's equally tragic for the kingdom of God. Talents, abilities, and opportunities are minimized because of declining health. Sometimes it can't be helped. Sometimes, however, it can be helped.

The turning point... Either we continue down the same unhealthy road or we find our turning point. Mine came when I hit the big double-nickel and realized I could either become proactive in maintaining better health and living the last half (okay, the last one-third... Call me Mr. Optimistic) of my life in the best possible shape I can be, or begin the dangerous slip-and-slide that would ultimately place me at greater risk for rising health concerns (not to speak of costs). I've made a proactive and healthy choice and I hope you will do the same.

Weight gain has never been that big of a problem for me. When you're 6'4" it's easy to hide it. However, when the scales hit 220+ and the waist-size approached 40", I knew it was time to slim down, eat better, exercise, and get disciplined and fit. And I have. I dropped twenty pounds (which doesn't sound like much until you pick up a twenty pound weight), eat more fruits and vegetables than ever, eliminate all sugar drinks, cut down on junk food, and stay committed to walking two to four miles daily. I go to bed earlier. I get up earlier. I don't watch the depressing national news any more. I feel better, have more energy, and enjoy a greater disposition about life than ever before. Last evening I walked three miles *in the rain* (at age fifty-five, you can do that). You may be thinking I don't have enough sense to come in out of the rain…Okay, you may be right. Then, again, I've always believed that everyone needs a good washing occasionally.

So what qualifies me to write a book like this? I'm not a doctor, nutritionist, or fitness expert. I'm a fifty-five year old student of history and human tendencies who has seen a lot of people come and go—and go way too early (as in "die"). Or who become sickly way too early. I think it's time someone addressed the issue in less than technical terms that people can understand—and with an underlying spiritual foundation. And that's the key. Most of the studies and books on the subject totally ignore this element of human existence. I believe we are the product of a loving God who created us to be the best we can be. It is the Creator and His design for us that should serve as our greatest and most powerful motivation for living healthy and long. The fact that you are still here living on *His* planet and breathing *His* oxygen obviously serves *His* purpose. Are you offering to Him (and through Him to others) the best you that you can give?

I'm not an alcoholic either, but can and do warn audiences of the dangers of that liquid drug and its aftereffects. And although I've never experimented with other drugs, I feel compelled to talk to kids about the consequences of addictive behavior resulting from wrong choices. It's not any different here.

The subject of this book is too serious an issue to keep pretending it is non-existent. Will some dismiss it (and me) and refuse to listen? Sure. It's like the man in the 1970s who said he was so tired of reading about the negative health effects of smoking that he decided to give up…*reading*. Many are like that today only with this addictive behavior. On the other hand, will some be motivated to take a second look in the mirror and make positive changes in their life because they know their life matters and affect others? I hope so.

You need to know something else, too. My wife, Julie, has struggled with weight issues for a long time. An emotional eater in the past, she has tried various diets in order to lose. And she has. And then re-gained. Many of you know the routine. It wasn't until a year ago that she took inventory, got serious about her issues, decided to own it, and do something about it. As an R.N. with a degree in Health Care Administration and over thirty years in the field of medicine, she knows the right answers to the questions. Knowledge is not her problem.

She met Gina Harris McDonald—the *Biggest Loser At Home Winner* (season 14) and Carter Hays (Gina's personal trainer in Franklin, Tennessee) at a local YMCA event. Gina's story was compelling and Carter's message was inspiring. When Valentine's Day rolled around, I gave Julie something absolutely unique: six weeks with Carter Hays. That was a first for me—and for her—*and for him!* Carter changed her outlook by helping Julie believe in herself and see who she really was. Instead of the quick fix and diet-of-the-month fad, he preached long-term life and mind change. On one occasion, Julie complained to Carter that she was sore from their last workout. He listened patiently. There was an awkward moment of silence when she finished, so she added, "Uh...I thought you would want to know." He replied with a smile, "Okay, now I know. Let's get to work."

By the way, Carter doesn't yell and scream like the *Biggest Loser* TV trainers (or, for that matter, like Sergeant Carter from the 1960s sitcom *Gomer Pyle USMC*). "That's nothing but entertainment drama," he says. The fact is; he's more likely to quote Scripture and encourage his clients with motivational thoughts and word-pictures. He is calm, kind, and focused. And his stories of success with his *Biggest Loser* clients as well as those that aren't are what draw others to him. He is a man of great compassion who helps hurting people cut through their excuses to discover the person God created them to be.

Carter Hays has agreed to help with this project and provide valuable insight from his years of experience in working with all kinds of people.

Julie has also agreed to open her life in these pages and become vulnerable. That isn't easy for her. She offers medical insight accompanied by the experience of one who has been there/done that and been there again. She knows all too well the painful struggle with food addiction. I love her with all my heart and am a willing participant in the journey with her. Count me as her biggest cheerleader.

Together, we want to be *your* cheerleader. No matter where you have been or are now, there is no better time to find your turning point than today. Tomorrow is too late and "someday" means never. Help with any addiction (yes, unhealthy eating can become an addiction) begins with an admission of a struggle. Pray about it and seek guidance from those qualified to give it. *You can* eat (notice I didn't say "diet"—that ugly four-letter word that should be rinsed from our mouths with soap) and *you can* move yourself to healthier habits, and in so doing, offer greater availability to the people God has placed in your life. After all, the biblical admonition to "love your neighbor as yourself" begins with...*loving yourself.* And my friend— *you* are worth it!

Are you ready for your personal *turning point?* If so, there are four very special (and very real!) people I want you to meet...

CHAPTER 1

Hidden Pain
Stories of Uncommon Courage

I waited patiently for the Lord; and He inclined to me and heard my cry. He brought me up out of the pit of destruction, out of the miry clay, And He set my feet upon a rock making my footsteps firm. (Psalm 40:1-2)

Andrew

Andrew is passionate about his journey. A thirty-five-year-old successful syndicated radio producer on Music Row in Nashville, Andrew's turning point came on February 6, 2008 when a friend who had been on NBC's *The Biggest Loser* Season Four pointed him to trainer Carter Hays. Andrew weighed 400 pounds, couldn't see his feet and couldn't run twenty yards. "Dude," his friend pleaded, "You have to get there." He did. Andrew well remembers the day he walked into the gym for the first time. "I felt everyone was looking at me," he said. "But I kept telling myself one thing—these people will never see me bigger than I am today." He faced his fears and changed his life.

His story is compelling.

"I was an emotional eater and became addicted to food. It was instant gratification followed by instant depression. When I went home feeling good, I rewarded myself with food. When I went home feeling bad, I looked for food as a fix. It wasn't uncommon for me to stop at McDonald's on the way home and eat a pre-dinner meal of a Double Quarter Pounder, two Double Cheeseburgers, a McChicken sandwich, large fries and a large soft drink. I then went home and ate my mother's cooking like I hadn't eaten all day. In fact, McDonald's became my secret place. Sometimes I would spend as much as twelve dollars on the $1 menu. I was an addict. While the crack addict has to go to the ghetto to get his fix, my fix was waiting for me on every street corner."

Sadly, he isn't alone. Fortunately, Andrew decided to take ownership.

"It's my fault I was fat. Today, it's my fault that I've lost 150 pounds. Neither has happened by accident. It took me a long time to get into the shape I was in and a long time to lose it. In fact, it took nine long and hard months to lose the first one hundred pounds. The office supply store, Staples, has ruined the world with their 'Easy Button'. We are so conditioned to think we can order weight loss as easy as we order food over the phone. That's not reality. In fact, there is no such thing as a successful diet. It doesn't exist. I watch the commercials and laugh when I see products claiming you can shake stuff on your food that will cause you to lose weight. They make it look so easy. You would think we would be smarter than that."

Sadly, many aren't.

"I've had to change everything I do and every way I used to think. I had to learn how to use food as fuel rather than as entertainment and comfort. For example, I had to learn that when I walk into a grocery store it's essential that I shop on the outside isles where the fruits and vegetables are located and stay away from the junk in the middle isles. And soda…don't even get me started talking about that. I had to learn that soda is the worst thing you can put into your body. And accountability…I had to make myself accountable 150%! There were so many things I had to learn."

Andrew is no longer into excuses nor does he seek sympathy. It wasn't always that way. Growing up in Topeka, Kansas, his childhood was fraught with hardship. Raised without a dad, his mother and older sister babied him. To fill his emotional void, he turned to food to fix the hurt. He also turned to humor. "I was the fat and funny guy," he explained. "Truth is; I just wanted to be normal, play sports, and take a girl on a date." He had plenty of girl friends, but never a girl *friend*. "Sometimes I stared at a guy and thought that I would like to wear pants like that and be able to tuck *my* shirt in."

Today he does. Andrew has lost 140 pounds and gone from a 4X to a more normal XL (which fits his frame). His secret is no secret. "I am just like you. I have a job. I have a family. Yet because I am a food addict, I must continually face my addiction. That's why my daily routine includes three non-negotiables: (1) drink water only, (2) eat real food, and (3) exercise forty-five minutes each day. No excuses."

It's not easy for him. He is smart enough to know that he isn't done just because he has lost the pounds. It's not like he started a diet, got some exercise, and then returned to "normal." It doesn't work that way. Obesity experts will tell you that losing weight is hard while keeping it off is even harder. That's why Andrew has a new "normal."

Andrew's new "normal" is to leave home before dawn each day and commute the hour into downtown Nashville. He works all morning until lunch. Then while others head for the nearest fast-food fare, Andrew makes the twenty minute drive south to the Franklin suburb where he attends an 11:00 AM "boot camp" workout with Carter before returning to work. On the day we met for a post-workout grilled chicken salad, Andrew confessed that he had "messed up" that morning and forgotten to pack his gym bag for his daily routine. "No excuses," he said. He merely stopped by a nearby sports store, bought what he needed, and never missed a beat. "I will never go back to where I was," he said. "But I know what I have to do to stay where I am."

Andrew's motto is: "You will never be as fat as you are today." And today he is passionate about using his life-change to help others. "I see a person who is obese and I see the person he/she is inside. And I know I can help that guy." He goes on, "I'm not a doctor. I don't have a degree attached to my name. I'm not a personal trainer. I'm just a fat guy who decided to change his life. And my message is simple: If I can do it, so can you!"

Andrew then leaned in with this poignant message—"You can't help those, however, who won't help themselves." He then added, "I only wish others could experience the feeling you get of losing and living."

Andrew found his turning point. It wasn't one and done for him, but a continued discipline of life-change. "I will always struggle with food addiction," he explained. Indeed, he will. Fortunately for him, he made the decision to do something about it. "February 6, 2008" was the day my life changed and I'm not looking back."

I have never met anyone with a greater passion for living.

Kate

Kate is a 38-year-old up-state New Yorker transplanted in the south. At 5'2", she exudes self-confidence with a spitfire personality and an endearing contagious smile. It hasn't always been that way.

Kate was not overweight as a child. In fact, she was quite athletic all the way through college. A fierce competitor, she was determined to be the best at whatever sport challenged her. In high school, it wasn't uncommon for her to practice soccer several hours each day. In college she not only practiced soccer for hours, but would often run an extra three miles *after* practice. "Coaches always liked me," she said. "Every team has a few players with heart and I was always one of those players."

She craved approval—from coaches, teammates, family, and friends. "My dad left our family when I was six years old," she said with a sigh. "My mother was always there for me and we were very close, though not having my dad around had an adverse effect on my life. I was hurt as a child, which turned into unresolved anger as an adult. I didn't know it at the time, but I became an emotional eater—turning to food rather than dealing with the conflict in my heart and head." A co-dependent personality emerged. "I became the quintessential peacemaker," she confided. "I had yet to learn that there is a big difference between loving people and allowing them to manipulate me."

Happily married at age 22, she got a job in corporate America, worked to pay bills, and slowly began to lose her healthy focus. She stopped exercising. She ate more. "French fries, pizza, ice-cream, you name it," she reminisced. "Before I knew it, I was carrying ten extra pounds. Then twenty. Then thirty. Sure, the weight bothered me, but I didn't think it was a big deal, until..." She paused before continuing. "Until the day my brothers took me aside, looked me in the eye, and asked, 'What's wrong?'" Kate's initial ten extra pounds had multiplied until the day of her brotherly intervention when she weighed 220 pounds. Something was wrong and obviously so.

As a young athlete, Kate could burn up the calories. Now, as a married working adult, she no longer had the time to do so. Or thought she didn't. And by the time her brothers intervened, she had become the master at social eating. "Chips and salsa became my weakness," she confessed. "Every time I turned around, there was another gathering and more junk to eat. I then found myself going home and snacking even more…"

Still young enough to be athletic, she looked in the mirror and said, "I've got this!" She bought a treadmill and began working out although she couldn't seem to get below the magical "170" line.

When she and her husband moved to Nashville in 2004, her diet and workouts remained rather yo-yo. There would be weight loss followed by weight gain. "My epiphany moment came when I turned thirty-one," she explained. "I had to ask myself the question: "Do I want to spend my 30s like I spent my 20s? And the answer was a resounding, 'No!'"

In 2006 she trained for a half-marathon. "I was a size 18 and still around 200 pounds," she explained. I worked hard, reduced food consumption to 1200 calories per day and eventually the weight started coming off. I went from 200 to 175 and then to 150 and as low as 133. I took my mile run from fifteen minutes to thirteen and finally to eight. I was back to where I needed to be. And then…then I gained it all again."

In 2011 she saw Hannah Curlee from Season 11 of *The Biggest Loser* mention Carter Hays on Twitter and mentioning his Boot Camp that she attended regularly. "Hannah had lost 120 pounds on the show and was looking great. She was from Nashville—also my hometown—so I contacted Carter and he invited me to come try out his Boot Camp" (a 45-minute group workout). By 2011, however, Kate's weight was still 200+ pounds. "The idea of working out with Hannah and the others was humiliating. Here I was, a former athlete and now…" In the coming days, her muscles would not hurt near as much as her pride. The former high school and college athlete who was used to being first was now last.

After a couple months, she sustained an injury, stopped going, and started running to lose the rest of the weight. In 2012 she lost down to 163. "I was looking and feeling better," she beamed enthusiastically. It wasn't long, however, until the stress of work and daily busyness put her back on the yo-yo. She gained back 50 pounds. So, in January, 2013, when the scale tipped 211 pounds, she went back to Boot Camp and made herself accountable. "I kept telling myself, 'Stop being afraid' and 'Just do your best.'" And while she found all kinds of excuses to quit, she didn't.

In May of 2013, Kate attended "Unleash the Champion"—a spring weeklong retreat in the Tennessee countryside. With talks by nutritionists, former *Biggest Loser* contestants, and with emphasis on how the body was designed by God to work properly, it comprised much more than a physical challenge. Participants were motivated to commit to a thirty-day countdown challenge. In fact, they were given assignments like—

- Take a quiet walk with God

- Write down the words to a song that moves you and then tell why

- Read a Psalm from Scripture and write in your own words what God is saying to you

- Describe on paper how you are fearfully and wonderfully made

"The problem for me," she said, "was the cost. But I decided I was worth it and needed this to change my life perspective." It did.

Kate has laid down a personal gauntlet. She challenged herself to attend Boot Camp for one year. No excuses. "I determined to go six days a week." Earlier in the year she met Gina Harris McDonald, an attorney from Birmingham, who had come to Nashville to train for the "at home" prize of Season 14 of *The Biggest Loser* (Gina would go on to win the prize in the season's finale). "She encouraged me so much. I thought—if she can do this three times a day, I can do it at least once a day."

All of this has left Kate feeling awesome about life. "I learned that I had to rid myself of all negative self-talk and that if I was to continue to be an encourager of others, I had to start encouraging myself as well." She laughed sheepishly. "People have even given me a new nickname—'Joy!'"

Kate made the decision to quit looking over her shoulder. "Knowing I had been an emotional eater, I asked God to help me. I had to learn that I have a purpose and that I am worth it. I have finally become that person."

Kate gets up every morning at 4:15 to attend the 5:00 Boot Camp. "I used to say I wasn't a morning person, but learned that it was nothing more than an excuse." She removed the words "I can't" from her vocabulary. "I've learned *I can* get up early and *I can* work out for 45 minutes and *I can* do this." She doesn't have much time for TV in her evenings now as she chooses, instead, to go to bed early. She makes better food choices. Her motto has become: *If you believe it, you can achieve it.* She then turned somber and said, "I so want to help others. I see overweight people and my heart goes out to them because that was me. And I want to say to them, 'You can do this! *You can do this!*'"

If it is more blessed to give than to receive (and it is), then Kate will be blessed. She has become the giver.

Michelle

Engaging. Energetic. Embracing. Those were the words Julie used to describe Michelle after our two hour meeting. Truthfully, she is all of that and more. To look at her one would never know her story and the struggles of her past. When it comes to stories, she has one. When it comes to struggles, hers have been epic. If anyone ever stepped up to the plate with two strikes against them, it was Michelle. Amazingly, she made the decision to move beyond her past and embrace her present with positive determination. She had one strike left and...she hit it out of the park. Her story is as inspiring as it is emotional.

Born and raised as a child in Springfield, Ohio, Michelle's memories of the first eight years of life are relatively happy ones although she never knew her real dad. When her mother's struggles with alcohol and drugs surfaced with a vengeance, her life took a tragic turn. From age eight to ten, Michelle went to eight different schools. She and her mother slept in shelters. They slept in the car. Men would come and go. "I believe she loved me, but Mom made some very bad choices. Sadly, I came to realize that I was not her first priority."

Her mother knew a family in Knoxville, Tennessee who agreed to take Michelle until her mother could get back on her feet. She never did. "I still remember meeting them at an Arby's where we unloaded suitcases and sacks from one car to the next. And that was it. I was never formally adopted but came to consider them my parents. I would still visit Mom on holidays and school breaks, but it became less and less."

Michelle knew that if she was going to break free from her past, she would have to do it on her own. And she did. She put herself through college—first at UT Knoxville and then at Tennessee Wesleyan where she graduated from their nursing program. By her early twenties she was balancing work, school, and a new marriage. Describing herself as "pudgy" as a child, Michelle began slowly putting on weight. "I seemed to gain about ten pounds each year," she said. "Not a lot, but the years—and the weight—started adding up." She found herself on the yo-yo road of weight loss, weight gain, and loss again. When she walked across the stage to receive her Masters Degree she weighed 225 pounds.

After moving to Nashville for graduate school, Michelle and her husband reached out and opened their home to an eight-year-old little girl. Less than a year later, they did the same thing again—this time embracing a three-year-old boy who desperately needed a home. The newly formed family of four crowded into their small 900 square foot apartment. Both children had special needs and represented unique challenges to the family. Michelle's life was full—in more ways than she could count.

Soon afterwards she was diagnosed with PCOS (Polycystic Ovary Syndrome) –a hormone disorder that affects fertility. It's a condition that affects approximately 5-10% of women of child-bearing age. It also makes it difficult to lose weight. "I believe God wanted us to adopt before we ever struggled with fertility," she said. "Adoption was our Plan A before there ever was a Plan B. In that sense, we give Him all the glory." That's Michelle—and it gives you some insight into the incredible person she is.

With a husband, two children, and a new career as a Nurse Practitioner, Michelle had been busy taking care of everyone except herself. She kept thinking of the verse in Hebrews 12:1—"lay aside every encumbrance..." Michelle's weight was her encumbrance. "I felt like God wanted to use me in different ways, but I knew the weight was an issue. I knew I had to get it off." Yet her insecurities were overwhelming. "All the junk in my past made it hard to move forward. I was so used to pleasing everyone else that I actually felt guilty of valuing myself."

She began watching Season 11 of the *Biggest Loser* and the journey of sisters Olivia Ward and Hannah Curlee. When they later posted a blog announcement of a retreat in middle Tennessee, Michelle went for it. "Just show up! Just show up!" she kept telling herself. She did show up and continues to show up. "I still struggle with admission issues," she confessed. "But I made the decision to own this and do something about it."

Michelle is slowly learning that the best way to be there for others (including her own family) is to take care of herself. She has learned that such an investment isn't selfish, but is, in fact, the very opposite. "You have to understand how hard this is for me, not only psychologically, but physically. I was never an athlete and never did sports. I never pushed myself. That is, until now." She also knew she had to draw closer to God. "As a nurse practitioner, knowledge and information is not my problem. What *is* my problem is the busyness of my life and the need to sit down, find moments of calm, and come to believe in myself."

She decided that food would not be her battle. She's worked hard and has lost 60 pounds. "I want to challenge myself with realistic goals—not to slip into a size 4, but to continue to keep physically fit by running a half marathon, building muscle, and letting my body figure out what a healthy weight will be rather than a number defined by the scale."

I asked Michelle what she would tell others attempting to climb similar mountains of hardship when it comes to weight-loss. "Three things," she said. "First, just show up! You have to start somewhere. Second, quit trying to figure everything out. I've learned that commitment breeds confidence and confidence breeds more commitment. Create a positive cycle that can be turned to your advantage. Third, do the best you can. As a Type A personality I had to accept that my best is good enough. And that's hard for me. I have a tendency to go too far, seek perfection, and live in the extreme. Yet it was my tendency towards perfection that kept me from starting in the first place. I had to make the decision to let it go..."

When I asked about excuses, she laughed. "I was the queen of excuses. And I had a million of them. Still do. Look, I have a husband who works full time as an accountant (over half the year he has to work overtime), two special needs kids—most weeks they have six therapy and tutoring appointments we must keep, and a part time job of my own. I can find excuses all day long to not take care of me." Instead, she found ways to be creative. On days she exercises with her group, she gets up at 4:30 in the morning. "If I want to make it happen, I have to make it happen. So, I make it happen. Believe me when I say I would much rather pull up the covers and sleep in. But I can't. I have to do this for me so I can be there for them." On days, for example, when she takes her kids to the park, she makes playtime fun time for them and exercise time for herself. "I'll race the kids down the street or run around and play with them like crazy," she smiles. "And they love it."

"Yes, I have a past, but I decided I don't have to continue down that path. I have a future, too, and I want it to be the very best. With God as my strength, I know it will be."

Engaging. Energetic. Embracing. Michelle has learned from her past, embraces her present, and smiles at her future. An incredibly busy wife and mom, she has found the secret to serving others: value self. It's something she's had to learn and, in some ways, it will always be a struggle for her. But she has made tremendous progress. Here is a woman who could easily play the popular blame game. She refuses. She has chosen to take responsibility for who she is and makes herself accountable in order to attain what she wishes to become. And instead of taking, she gives back.

It is said that most people miss out on life because they live in the *someday*. Michelle has embraced the truth that *someday* is either right now or never. She has chosen to make it right now.

Tracy

Tracy is hitting his stride. He's also hitting a life milestone—turning the big 5-0. He's a hard-charging people person; a successful businessman in a tough and competitive field: real estate. His phone rings constantly. His work hours are all over the chart. He and his wife, Sharon, have raised four girls; two are now in their early twenties while the twins are sixteen. He was recently appointed a church elder where his family worships. Tracy is busy—sometimes crazy busy.

He is also concerned about his health, sees mistakes he's made in the past, and is working hard to turn things around. This is a turning point moment for him and he knows it.

"I have to set a better example for my girls," he said over coffee. "I'm not really sure we taught them how to eat right. In fact, during their growing up years, like a lot of families, we tended to eat high fat meals that included lots of bread and butter. And, like others, we had a rule: 'Clean your plate.'" He went on... "I remember once Sharon had beets as a vegetable with the meal. She loves beets. I don't like them at all. And that night we learned that the girls didn't like them either. But rule are rules. So, I ate mine. Then we waited for the girls to eat theirs. All I remember was that supper lasted over two hours that night," he said laughing. "Seriously, we thought the 'always clean your plate' rule was the right thing..."

"And we rewarded the girls with food. Good grades, for example, would merit a special evening treat at Dairy Queen or Sonic. Food was fun. Sweets were the reward." He thought a moment and added, "I guess we could have made some changes by rewarding them differently. Then, again, buying ice cream was a lot cheaper than taking them shopping for new clothes."

His next question was one about which many parents struggle. "What now?" And "how do we fix it?"

Tracy and Sharon decided to "fix it" by fixing themselves and setting a better example. "I decided it was time for a change and that change started with me." He went on to say that he was committed to doing things differently for himself—and for his family.

Growing up as a boy in the country, Tracy was on the heavy side in grade school. "It wasn't too bad," he said, "although I remember hating to go shopping with momma and buying those 'Husky jeans.'" He remained on the pudgy side until about the fifth or six grades when he started to slim down. His chores helped. "The older I became the more chores I had. I would either be helping in the garden, or clearing fence rows and hauling hay." By the time he graduated high school and went off to college he was 5'8" and weighed a slim 160 pounds. "I enjoyed college-life," he said. "And the best parts about college? Pizza! I discovered pizza! Do you know how many pieces of pizza I could put away?" he said with a laugh.

It was after he married that the weight started increasing and eventually took him from 160 to 213 pounds. "I liked to eat," he admitted. "I did a lot of traveling in those days and I pampered myself. On business trips the company paid for my meals and those of clients and I went to some really good places." He continued, "I mean, everyone else was ordering this huge meal; what was I supposed to do, eat a salad?"

"I've always been a sauce guy," he confessed. "If the food wasn't covered with some kind of cheese sauce, crème sauce, etc., I wasn't interested. In fact, you could probably pick the worst thing on a restaurant menu and that's what I ate." He went on. "I also worked for a company back then that made pumps for soft drink dispensers. As a result, we had one of those machines at work with all the free soft drinks you could drink. After all, someone needed to test the product. Let's just say I was quite the team player," he grinned. "Come to think of it, almost everyone who worked there was heavy. We drank soft drinks all day long."

At one point Tracy had to have a physical. The doctor's wife, who happened to be a family friend, looked at the numbers from his blood work and exclaimed, "You are a walking heart attack!" His cholesterol had reached 285."

"Soon afterwards, I ran into a business associate on a trip out to California and this guy had always been heavy. When I saw him that day, he had lost a bunch of weight. When he told me about the success he had with the Atkins Diet, I couldn't get to a bookstore fast enough. I bought the book, read it, and decided to go for it." It worked. And fast. In nine months he was down to 155 pounds and his cholesterol was in the normal range. He maintained it for a while and then started gaining it all back. "A little bread won't hurt me," he reasoned. "A little dessert will be okay." Six months later he was right back where he started.

Eventually he came up with a diet plan of his own: *The Tracy Diet*. *The Tracy Diet* was simple. He would eat whatever he wanted from Thanksgiving through Christmas. Come January he would cut back. "That worked until the warmer weather hit and all the cookouts started," he chuckled. "And I had to have homemade ice cream!" And when Halloween rolled around, someone had to help the girls "sort" through all that candy. "Pretty soon, it was back to Thanksgiving and the process repeated." He admits to loosing 300 pounds—thirty pounds ten different times! "Talk about a yo-yo..."

He was with a loan officer friend named Marty on the way back from lunch one day when they saw a sign advertising a gym. Tracy said half-joking, "We ought to go and take care of this [weight]." He never expected Marty to take up the challenge. He did. He remembers well the date: December 31, 2011. They walked into the gym, got a trainer, and made themselves accountable.

"I would not do what I am supposed to do without him," Tracy acknowledged. "If the trainer is standing beside me and I'm supposed to do twenty pushups, I do twenty push-ups. On the other hand, if he's not there the day I'm supposed to do my workout and the discomfort starts when I hit fifteen pushups, I stop at fifteen. It's the same with the stairs. I always finish when he's with me. He's challenges me every step of the way..."

Tracy hasn't looked back. In addition to his three-day-a-week workout with a trainer, he runs on the other days with friends from church. And he gets up early. "I'm not naturally a morning person, but on the days I run, I get up at 5:00 and meet the others at 6:00. On the days I meet my trainer, I'm at the gym by 7:30." He has to. By 9:00 in the morning his phone starts ringing non-stop. "If I waited until evening to run or work out, well...something always happens and I'll end up not going. I look at it like saving money. If you don't save the money first, you'll figure out a way to spend it. It's not any different. So I exercise first thing."

He makes a smoothie every morning. "Strawberry and peaches with yogurt and some protein powder." Or maybe he'll have fresh coffee and a banana along with some chocolate protein powder mixed with almond milk. After he works out he downs a protein shake.

He enjoys describing the breakfast he had before his first trip to the gym. "It was our daughter Allison's birthday. We went to Mimi's to celebrate and I had waffles stuffed with crème cheese, scrambled eggs, bacon, topped off with a sweet muffin. I left the restaurant and went to work out. Let's just say it's not a routine I ever did again or would ever recommend," he said laughing.

"I enjoy working out, but only if I have someone to do it with," he said. "It's all about accountability." He added, "It's the same with running… I'll run three or four miles alone and quit. If I'm with others, I'll always go farther."

Tracy admits he feels better than ever. He built up his stamina and ran in a 15K race for Special Kids last March. He's planning on running a half marathon this fall and a full marathon in December to benefit St. Jude's Children's Research Hospital in Memphis. At 175 pounds he feels great. He works out, watches what he eats, and is committed to staying healthy. "I used to go to Olive Garden and order their Italian Sampler meal. That was my absolute favorite. I would eat the whole thing along with salad and three or four breadsticks. I don't do that anymore. I may still go to Olive Garden occasionally, but I'll get a smaller portion and something much healthier."

I asked if there were a couple non-negotiables he would recommend. "Two things," he said. "First, you have to have a trainer," he said with a look of seriousness. "And get a good one—one that fits you. For example, Sharon has a different trainer than I do. And that's okay. Second, you have to get it in your head that you can do this. No excuses. You have to be committed." He went on, "I've done this now for a year and a half and it has changed my life. It's not a fad; in fact, I look forward to it. Listen, I work a lot of hours and go full speed and used to tire easily. Not any more. I have more energy than ever."

Tracy has a big birthday just around the corner. He's already given himself and his family the best present any half-century guy can have: his health.

Summary

Real people. Real change.

In one of Charles Schultz's Peanuts comic strips, Charlie Brown says, "I think I've discovered the secret of life—you just hang around until you get used to it." I am convinced that is the way most people live. They just get used to it. The problem is that none of us improve by simply living. You have to be intentional about it. I hate to tell you but motivation is not going to strike you like lightning. You have to make the decision to change. And while you cannot change your destination overnight, you can change your direction. But you have to "want to."

It's been said that you cannot change your life until you change something you do every day. Life change is a daily endeavor. Each of these four people changed something they did every day. They made a decision to be proactive. They made a decision to stop with the excuses. They made a decision to become accountable.

They made a decision to be proactive. Each of them confessed to us their weaknesses toward food. Yet each of them equally acknowledged the greater power they felt when they consciously thought through their food decisions and made better choices. And each of them can point to the exact day they made the decision to stop blaming, take responsibility for their lives, and create positive momentum. You never forget your turning point.

They made a decision to stop with the excuses. These are all busy people with the potential for dozens of excuses—the same kind all of us can make. Yet they found a way. If it means getting up early in the morning, they get up early in the morning. If it means working out during their lunch break, they work out during their lunch break. If it means sacrificing financially for the good of their health, they sacrifice financially for the good of their health. If it means saying "No" to certain foods and peer pressure, they say "No" to certain foods and peer pressure. What all of them have found is this: what they have given up doesn't measure up to re-gaining their health and becoming the person they always wanted to be.

They made a decision to become accountable. Interestingly enough, this common denominator kept surfacing. They realized if they were going to climb the mountain toward better health, they needed help. The accountability factor with each of them was a non-negotiable. It reminds me of the verse in Ecclesiastes: "Two are better than one…For if either of them falls, the one will lift up his companion. But woe to the one who falls when there is not another to lift him up" (4:9-10). That's accountability.

True, there are some situations that require a little tweaking that you can do on your own. Some people are self-starters and self-motivators. Good for them. However, they are in the minority. Most need help and help means accountability. Accountability costs and some aren't willing to pay the price in terms of money, time, overcoming peer pressure, embarrassment, energy and just plain old-fashioned sweat. Yet everything worthwhile comes with a price. And you get what you pay for.

One final thing impressed us about each of them. They were passionate about regaining their health and encouraging others toward the same. If enthusiasm is caring—really caring about something worthwhile—these four have captured its essence. You cannot spend time with them and come away depressed. They made a decision to turn their life around. They worked hard. They remain a work in progress. And…they wanted to share their stories.

They have.

If each of them could do it, so can you.

CHAPTER 2

Food
The Unspeakable Addiction

...for by what a man is overcome, by this he is enslaved.
(2 Peter 2:19b)

We are eating ourselves to disease and death—*literally!* Yet because of its sensitivity and prevalence, it remains the "untouchable" subject. We laugh about it. We smile as we leave the potluck dinner and nudge the preacher, "Sure hope the sermon tonight isn't on gluttony..." Wink. Wink. Seriously, when was the last time you heard a sermon on gluttony? I can't remember any. Maybe we need to hear some. Solomon warned about those with "great appetites" (Proverbs 23:2). Paul talked about people whose "god is their appetite" (Philippians 3:19). And when His detractors called Jesus a "glutton" (Luke 7:34), it wasn't a compliment (it also wasn't true).

"Whether, then, you eat or drink or whatever you do, do all to the glory of God" (1 Corinthians 10:31). Are we eating and drinking to our gluttony or to God's glory? Given the health crisis of our day, it's a critical (and valid) question.

We have to start telling the truth. We're so conditioned to be politically correct and socially sensitive, that we end up skirting the whole food-health-overweight issue. That must change.

Food Addiction—*Really?*

Society and the medical profession have long understood the addictive nature of alcohol, nicotine, and drugs of various kinds. Only in more recent years, however, has education led to our understanding and acceptance that *food* can also become a trigger for addictive behavior. Fat, salt, and sugar (the perfect storm of junk food) can trigger reward responses in our brains that make cravings hard to ignore.

When substances are taken into the body regardless of their potential for harm or taken in excess of reasonable need, that substance is said to be abused. Those who abuse themselves in such a way are addicts. An addict is simply one who becomes dependent upon certain substances that give them a "high" either physiologically or mentally. In the case of food, it involves the compulsive, abnormal, and excessive craving for food to fill a void in their life.

Food addicts come in all shapes, sizes, races, as well as in both genders. They may be overweight, underweight, or appear to be normal in weight. The obese individual suffers the most humiliation due to his/her excess weight. The results are there for everyone to see. On the other hand, the underweight individual may hide his/her eating disorder even though it is equally abusive. It is quite common for the bulimic individual to binge eat and then induce vomiting, take laxatives, or exercise compulsively in order to prevent weight gain. Anorexia is another eating disorder that is more common in teenagers and involves such a fear of weight gain that the individual doesn't eat enough to promote reasonable weight and health. Then, again, the person of normal weight may be so obsessed with food that it drives their life to the point of neurosis. They are constantly stressing over what to eat (or not eat), how much they weigh, and counting calories compulsively. Sadly, these individuals cannot enjoy a simple single meal. They have no concept of Solomon's wisdom involving contentment, life moderation, and satisfaction.

> Here is what I have seen to be good and fitting: To eat, to drink and enjoy oneself in all one's labor in which he toils under the sun during the few years of his life which God has given him for a reward. (Ecclesiastes 5:18)

Like any other addictive behavior, food addiction (in any form) involves a loss of control. This person understands that their habits are harmful, but continues the destructive pattern anyway. Suffering from depression, low self-esteem, or plain old loneliness, the individual eats to feel better. However, the "high" quickly disappears and gives way to feelings of guilt (which leads to more depression). And even though the addict promises himself/herself they will stop, they turn once more to the same eating patterns in order to feel better. It is a vicious cycle.

Emotional Eating

Many overeaters over indulge because it fills a void that is much deeper and bigger than the one in their stomach. In other words, they feed their feelings. Some studies report that 75% of overeating is caused by emotions. We even have a new phrase that has come into the American vocabulary to describe such: *comfort foods*. These are foods that are…well…*comfortable*. They lift us up when we are down. Someone described them as "comfort food Kryptonite"—they make us feel "super" (the "super" doesn't last very long). Comfort foods that give us the most comfort are usually things like ice cream, potato chips, candy, cookies, and chocolate. We eat to manage our emotions and because we like the "feel good" sensation we attain, we eat much more than we should.

The problem is this: the body doesn't know what to do with non-nutritional and fun foods. For example, the stomach digests an apple and knows exactly what to do with it—sending hundreds of vitamins and nutrients to all the right places. On the other hand, when we eat processed chips, suddenly the body asks, "Uh…okay…what am I supposed to do with this?" And because it doesn't know what to do with it, it just stores it away for a rainy day (usually on your hips!).

Elimination isn't always the answer (although sometimes it is) as much as moderation. The problem isn't that we eat a scoop of ice cream occasionally or a few potato chips, but that we eat too many of them. We get way too much *comfort* from *comfort* foods (most of which don't qualify as real food at all). Then, again, we've been conditioned to equate feelings with food. What does a parent offer a child who is sad? Usually it's a special (and sugary!) treat. "Here, Johnny, this sugar will make you *feel* better!"

Learning how to deal with our feelings without food is a whole new experience for many of us.

It is here I must call a "time out" and offer a balanced perspective. When someone asks, "Isn't most eating emotional?"—I would have to answer, yes. If that isn't the case, then I'm at a loss to explain why we spend so much time finding food, preparing it, and then sharing it with family and friends. While our bodies were designed by God to use food as fuel for survival, there is more going on each day than mere physiology.

Our culture has long used food as a bonding mechanism for bringing people together. We use food to mark both sad and happy occasions. Even after Uncle Joe's funeral, the entire family heads back to the Uncle Joe homestead to kill the fatted calf (or at least to devour ham and potato salad) and swap funny stories. You cannot divorce food from social (emotional) gatherings. It's for this reason that diets don't work very well. Each of us live social (emotional) lives in which we interact with others—many times around food. Birthday parties, going out for lunch with a friend, eating pizza on Friday nights, holiday dinners; you can't escape it. In each of these shared experiences there is pleasure (emotion). That isn't always a bad thing. However, when we cross the line of moderation and begin to use food consistently as our means of escape, we're heading down a very unhealthy road.

People look for something to fill the hole in their soul. It's why some become alcoholics while others become workaholics. Each is finding a way to cope, fill the emptiness, and escape the pain—if only for the moment. Some escape by turning to recreation and entertainment in the extreme. Some even turn to "church busyness"—anything to escape. And some turn to food. Like the drug addict getting a temporary fix, food becomes the legal and easy "high" that many find. That's what I mean by *emotional eating*. It may not be so much what you are eating as much as what's eating you.

Julie's Hiding Place

Listen as my wife describes her emotional eating past.

> Emotional eating for me was a momentary escape from hurt, anger, discouragement, guilt, pain (or whatever else was on my

"plate" at the moment). By eating, you suddenly feel free from the "weight" that is trapped inside. Ironically, that moment is actually destroying you, but the need to escape overcomes all rational thinking.

Most emotional eaters do so in secret or when alone because of the façade we build about how we handle our baggage. To own up to our secret only brings more pain, discouragement, and guilt.

People come to this escape for various reasons. Perhaps their childhood was one where food was the reward given for good behavior or accomplishments and a way to enjoy parental approval. It could be the result of emotional trauma in a variety of relationships. Whatever the reason, food becomes a solace that cannot be supplied anywhere else.

I recall as a little girl visiting my grandparents in Ohio. My maternal grandfather was very special to me. He gave me his undivided attention on those visits and would play "Beauty Shop" with me as I placed his thinning gray hair in all kinds of silly styles. On those visits, we would make a "just us" trip to Woolworths in downtown Portsmouth. That store was a child's happy place. Besides the toys, there was a soda fountain—you know, the one with the shiny agua blue stools upon which you would sit and be served by waitresses with white uniforms and pointed hats.

Papaw and I would sit on those stools and order "pop" (as it was called in that part of the country) along with a slice of lemon pie (his favorite). By then I already had my bag of M&M's that he had purchased for me from the counter where all the candy is behind glass and delivered in white bags via a big silver scooper. As he ate his pie, he would smile and say, "Now Julie, don't tell your Mamaw about this because I'm not supposed to have it" (he was diabetic). "Okay!" I would reply while sipping my soft drink through a straw and grabbing another handful of my favorite chocolate candy. Life was grand!

The emotional high found in a similar bag of M&M's years later became quick and easily accessible. During that moment I felt good about myself...as if I was like everyone else who was "thin." Even before the purchase, I had talked myself into believing this was the best thing for me because I deserved it. After all, suffering in any way deserves a reward.

It was after the bag was empty that the guilt set in. Why did I do that? You quickly remove the nagging thoughts because you just aren't sure what to do about it anyway.

I found the cycle repeating itself as long as I tried carrying the baggage alone. Some may ask, "Aren't Christians supposed to let God carry their emotional baggage?" Yes—but to do so meant I would have to leave my secret and safe hiding place to give it to Him. I wasn't ready to do that (or so I thought). To leave my secret place would mean that not only would He see the junk in my life, but so would others. Ironically, others saw it anyway—every time they looked at me.

Emotional eating is best understood by those who have been there. On the other hand, those who haven't will not understand the struggle. What looks so simple to outsiders can become very complex when you're the one on the inside of the spin cycle trying to clean the junk from your mental attic. Some of you have taken this journey and you know exactly what this means. Emotional eating is what you do when you don't know what to do. It's quick. It's easy. It's a way to feel better about your private pain. As one person told me, "Food becomes your best and safest friend." Unfortunately, however, it doesn't fix the problem; it only masks it.

Using food from time to time as a comfort or a pick-me-up or to celebrate a special occasion isn't always a bad thing. However, if food becomes your primary coping mechanism to deal with stress, anger, loneliness, boredom, etc., you will find yourself in a very unhealthy situation. And I know you don't want that.

Suggestions for Coping

How can I fight off the urge to eat when I'm lonely or discouraged? Here are ten suggestions:

- Stick your iPod in your ear, strap on some new walking shoes and get moving. You don't have to obsess (or stress) about exercise or walk several miles, but you do have to move. So…move. It's better than sitting on the couch and…well, you know. Physical exercise will work wonders for your mood and energy levels. And your hips will thank you, too.

- Phone a friend and talk somewhere—other than the kitchen.

- Find a new comfort food—something healthy that you can snack on (preferably fruits, vegetables, and berries).

- Eliminate the junk from your fridge and pantry. I know you paid good money for that stuff, but if it's there—you'll eat it. Eliminate the temptation.

- Keep your water bottle handy. In fact, get a "cool" one—something that fits your personality—and drink God's beverage. It's been around for years and has never been improved upon. After all, when God designed your body, He made it 70% water. So replenish what He put in. Oh yeah, it has ZERO calories. Drink up. (Hint: Julie cuts fresh lemons and limes and adds them to the water pitcher we keep in the fridge. It gives cold water an extra "kick." Try it.)

- Take a hot bath, light some scented candles, get a cup of hot tea and lose yourself in a good book (this suggestion is probably gender specific).

- If you need a taste of cake, shrink the portion to three or four bites—just enough to get the pleasure. If it's ice cream, half a bowl and loaded up with fruit.

- Stop and think. Ask yourself: Is this really what I want to do? Write 1 Corinthians 10:31 ("Whether you eat or drink or whatever you do, do all to the glory of God") on a posted note and stick it on your fridge, in your car, or wherever it needs to be seen.

- Sleep. Sleep is an invaluable asset when it comes to mental alertness and recharging your body. One study from the University of Chicago concluded that the less sleep you get the more likely you are to overeat the following day. Since your success depends upon mental discipline, give your mind (and body) the edge it needs.

• Drink more water. Swallow and repeat.

My wife and I recently celebrated a special occasion at a favorite restaurant and decided to split a dessert. We usually don't have any so this was a treat. When the dessert came, we were in shock. We may have had two plates and two forks, but there was enough cake there to feed a multitude. We took our few bites and brought it home to reward our teenager. And he didn't eat it all. Some restaurants don't understand the word "moderation." In fact, most of them don't. Remember: you are in control of what goes into your mouth. And remember this, too: you can't outrun (or out exercise) your fork. But more about that later...

Did I say to drink more water?

Is Recovery Possible?

Like all other dangerous habits, eating disorders bring on a host of health-related consequences (obesity, diabetes, heart disease, greater cancer risk, sleep apnea, etc.). You don't have to be a part of the medical community to realize the obvious. Medicines and ambulatory aids may make us more mobile and keep us alive longer, but are we healthier, happier, and wiser? I don't think so.

Are there common-sense steps to recovery and reclaiming your life—so as to be more available for God and those He puts in your life? Yes! Please be advised, however, that the process of change will not be easy. Then, again, nothing worthwhile ever is. And this is worthwhile. We're talking about you as God's child becoming the person you were created to be. And you can do it.

However, if you've been using food for decades as your means of coping, those behavior patterns won't disappear overnight. You need a long-term action plan. Here goes...

1. Admission of the problem. As long as the food addict (or any other addict) lives in denial, recovery is not possible. That's why the first step for addiction recovery is the realization and acceptance of the problem. And why? Because it is impossible to solve a problem you do not think you have.

One needs only to ask a few simple questions to determine the reality of the problem.

- Do you eat when you feel down and depressed?

- Do you eat in secret or eat differently when in the company of others?

- Does food make you feel safe?

- Do you eat in excess? (Yes, an entire bag of chips, box of cookies, a two liter and super-sized helpings of junk food are in excess)

- Do you feel guilty after eating?

If you answer "Yes" to questions like these, you need to admit that a problem exists. Denying it won't make it go away. And excuses won't solve the problem either. I smiled at the line Dr. Mehmet Oz gave recently, "People say their weight is genetic. But people who are overweight also have overweight pets. That's not genetic." I don't think Dr. Oz is into excuses. And neither should you be.

Rhonda from Ohio knows the emotional struggle all-too-well…

I have fooled myself into thinking that it's acceptable to eat five pieces of pizza. I trick myself into thinking that a salad with fried chicken, bacon, cheese, croutons, and extra bleu cheese dressing is a healthy option. It's okay if I go to the fast-food Mexican restaurant at 11:00 PM for their self-proclaimed "4th meal" and eat nachos and tacos before bed. I can drink a 64 ounce Diet Coke a day but can't seem to find time to drink any water. Two bowls of cereal? No problem. Super-sized fries? Why not? Dessert after every meal? A necessity.

Denying myself things that I enjoy (and on some level may have an actual addiction) is not pleasant. It's not going to be easy. But if I want to reap the benefits of being a healthy person, I have a choice to make. I can stop putting garbage into my body every day and live longer and have a more comfortable life, or I can continue to deceive myself and pretend that the choices I make today aren't going to affect me down the road.

Rhonda finds comfort in *comfort* food. And it's slowly killing her. Yes, she has a choice to make and she's right that it won't be easy. But you must have a starting place and that starting place is admitting your struggles. And she has. Admission of the problem, however, doesn't solve it. The starting line is not the finish line.

2. It will require intense mental discipline. Any attempt to change habitual behavior will be met with strong mental resistance. Even though you want to become healthier, your mind will fight back. And it will be the hardest fight of your life. That's why the battle will be won (or lost) in the mind (and that's true regarding any temptation). Fix the mind and the body will follow. The Bible recognizes this truth. "All things are lawful for me, but not all things are profitable. All things are lawful, but I will not be mastered by anything" (1 Corinthians 6:12). Has food become your "master?" Peter writes, "...for by what a man is overcome, by this he is enslaved" (1 Peter 2:19). Has food "enslaved" you? Consider two more verses:

But I discipline my body and make it my slave...(1 Corinthians 9:27)

For as he thinks within himself, so is he. (Proverbs 23:7)

Both of these verses depict one who makes the decision to win the battle of the mind. And it is a battle you must win decisively and consistently. Just because you win the mind-war and make better health-choices today, doesn't mean you will tomorrow. In fact, Satan will redouble his efforts in order to re-claim you as his prisoner. This is a battleground that you must fight (and win!) daily.

3. Confess your struggles to your family. That's hard to do, because you may not be able to gauge their reaction. You fear they may second-guess you, be disappointed in you, judge you, listen to what you order from a menu, laugh at you, spy on you, or even speak words to discourage you from your decision to change your life. However, it is *your* life. Speak to them openly, calmly, and ask for their encouragement and prayers. They already know you have food issues, so own it.

4. Make yourself accountable. Any attempt to break the bonds of addiction (regardless of what type) must utilize accountability. You must empower others to hold you accountable and to whom you are responsible. And while it is important to confess your struggles to family members, it is equally important to embrace this reality check: **relatives and close friends don't qualify for accountability partners!** Family and friends don't usually work well in the accountability arena for one simple reason: they don't wish to be offensive and "hurt your feelings." They, after all, have the wonderful pleasure of living with you and/or around you and most of them will not be overly excited to upset your apple cart (or chocolate cart).

Here's the deal. If you're looking for pity, there are plenty of people who can offer that. Most of us, however, are fully capable of feeling sorry for ourselves without much assistance. Find someone trustworthy who will agree to tell you what you *need* to hear and not necessarily what you want to hear. These people aren't into pity parties or excuses. They are into truth, accountability, and responsibility.

That person may be a religious leader, physician, life coach, fitness trainer, or any number of qualified and responsible individuals. You may need to spend some money in order to use their resources. Spend the money. You are, after all, making a life investment on the front end. I've noticed that when people have a financial "buy-in," they are much more likely to take advice and coaching seriously.

The bottom line, however, is this: No one will help the food addict until the food addict helps himself/herself. It's up to you.

5. Get informed. In Bob Harper's book, *The Skinny Rules*, the popular *Biggest Loser* trainer states, "We are bombarded from every direction with health advice—about diet, nutrition, weight loss, exercise…Now add in the daily science and medical news, a lot of which sounds stunningly obvious (not being obese=good) or ridiculously counter to what we *thought* was correct (fruit juice=not so good), and you've got a jumbo case of Clutter Brain." He goes on to say that Clutter Brain happens when you get so much information that the mind becomes numb to processing and making reasonable sense from it. It happens. We are, after all, in the age of information overload.

There are tools available to help cut through the clutter and enable you to follow some common-sense rules of living. Harper's book is a great source. Carter Hays' book, *Discover Your Road to Divine Health*, has a section called, "Real People, Real Food, Real Simple" that is solid gold you can take to the bank. These guys are not only professional trainers but great communicators. They cut to the chase and tell it like it is in simple terms you can understand. Their books are not the only ones out there (there are hundreds!), but they are two I've read and have concluded that these guys "get it." Oh yeah, they aren't into excuses either.

The internet can also provide a wealth of information. But beware…as with anything on the web, your search shovel may turn up both good and bad. Be discerning.

6. Pray and seek God's help. Dependency upon food can best be broken when the individual recognizes they need divine assistance. The Creator is able to provide help and healing in all areas of human weaknesses. Exodus 15:26—"For I, the Lord, am your healer." And consider Psalm 40:1-2—

> I waited patiently for the Lord; and He inclined His ear to me and heard my cry. He brought me up out of the pit of destruction, out of the miry clay.

Who lifts us from the "miry clay?" God does. Some translations render this "the mud of the mire"—depicting one sinking deeper and deeper into the quicksand of despair. Maybe that's where you are or have been. Listen, God is concerned about your physical well-being just as he is concerned with everything else. He wants you to be fully alive, healthy, and happy—letting your light shine brightly before others. He wants you to be available as His servant in order to lift up others. He wants you to love your neighbor to the extent that you love (care for) yourself. He wants you to obey every part of His will, including caring for the one and only physical body He has provided. "Or do you not know that your body is a temple of the Holy Spirit who is in you, whom you have from God, and that you are not your own? For you have been bought with a price: therefore glorify God in your body" (1 Corinthians 6:19-20).

Seek Him daily. Engage a regimen of conversation that begins first with Scripture. It's been said that the quality of a conversation is often dictated by the one who starts it. So, let God initiate the conversation. The Bible, after all, is God speaking to us.

If you don't know where to start—try Psalms. Or James. Or maybe one of the biographical accounts of the life of Christ (Matthew, Mark, Luke, John). You don't have to read large portions or lengthy chapters. Read until a statement is made that addresses you and your need (if you are like me, you won't have to read far). Then STOP. Take a moment and savor the verse. Highlight it. Meditate on it. Then ask, "What is the Lord trying to tell me?"

Then bow your head in silent solitude and ask for wisdom, guidance, and help (and don't forget to be thankful for past victories and blessings). "But if any of you lacks wisdom, let Him ask of God, who gives to all generously…" (James 1:5). And is God capable of delivering? Consider—

> No temptation has overtaken you but such as is common to man; and God is faithful, who will not allow you to be tempted beyond what you are able, but with the temptation will provide the way of escape also, so that you may be able to endure it. (1 Corinthians 10:13)

> Now to Him who is able to do far more abundantly beyond all that we ask or think, according to the power that works within us… (Ephesians 3:20)

And when you pray, pray BIG! Pray boldly. Pray persistently. Ask and keep on asking. After all, you're talking to the Great "I AM"—the God who moves mountains, the "How Great Thou Art" God. Lay your burden on His shoulders. Seek His intervention. Praise Him for what He can do. Don't be afraid. Pray BIG.

Is God capable of delivering? Listen, if the God of the world can create this beautiful earth out of nothing, He is fully capable and completely competent to handle you and your troubles. Wrap your arms of faith around Him and ask Him to help you find your turning point. He will. And you can.

CHAPTER 3

We're Living Longer, but Are We Living Better?

*As for the days of our life, they contain seventy years,
or if due to strength, eighty years, yet their pride is but labor
and sorrow; for soon it is gone and we fly away.*
(Psalms 90:10)

Age happens. I hate to be the bearer of bad news, but you *are* getting older. The birthday card that reads, "You're not getting older, you're getting better," is certainly said in jest. The *bad* news is...age eventually catches up to all of us. The *good* news is...given modern-day advances in medicine, we are living longer. Consider the increase in the average American lifespan:

1900—47 years

1940—63 years

1980—73 years

2000—78 years

Okay, maybe this will make you feel better (then, again, maybe it won't). Here it is: if this rate of increase continues, by the year 3000 the average American will live to be 328 years old (kudos to a mathematician friend from Middle Tennessee State University for working out this calculation). Now that's a lot of birthday candles! And while we'll never put up

Methuselah-type numbers, that's still a long time to be around (even half that number—or a third—would be impressive). Think about it... You may need an extra wide-angle lens for your family reunion photos! After all, there's nothing quite like those great, great, great, great, great, great, great, great, great, great, great grandchildren!

Each sunrise and sunset is a reminder of the brevity of life. In the grand scheme of things, life on planet earth is a mere "vapor that appears for a little while and then vanishes away" (James 4:14). Each birthday brings the reminder that time is slipping away. And the birthdays only come faster and faster. There are, however, two facts of reality looking back at us in the mirror every morning: (1) most of us are living longer, but (2) most of us are not living better. *Why?*

Think about it... We have more health information at our fingertips (literally!) than ever before, yet are unhealthier than ever before. What this says is simple. Health care in twenty-first century America is a misnomer. It has been relegated to managed "sick care." We simply have the meds to manage the symptoms of our illnesses over longer periods of time. Besides, everyone knows insurance companies pay off in areas of sick care instead of well care. So, we are conditioned to wait until we are sick, see a doctor, get test results, obtain prescription drugs, and bill insurance. We then repeat the cycle. Proactive health care or managed sick care? We have it backwards.

Managed Mediocrity

One reason for the current medical mindset is that we've become accustomed to mediocrity—in everything. We have accepted average health, average jobs, average strength, average dreams, average you-name-it. We have become a society of "average" only because we've been told this is the way it has to be. *Really?* Carter Hays writes in the introduction of his book, "I suppose any discussion regarding our health and wellness should begin with a 'state-of-your condition' speech. I can tell you this: you were created to have abundant energy, imagination, creativity, muscular strength and endurance; to wake up refreshed, go to sleep tired, eat real food, love your life, love your neighbor, laugh a lot, cry a little, pray unceasingly, dream big dreams, look for challenges to overcome, and realize you can have all of this and more…or none of this." He's right. It's your choice. So why do we settle for less? Could it be because everyone else does? Thus the blind follow the blind (average begets average) and we all end up in the ditch called "mediocrity."

Think with me a moment. Is it possible to live your whole life from an entirely wrong perspective? Yes. I love the story told by several authors of the little boy who found an eagle's egg. Unable to reach the eagle's nest, he placed the egg in the nest of a prairie chicken. The result was predictable. The hen sat on the egg and it hatched alongside her baby prairie chickens. Here's the story…

> All his life, the eagle (thinking he was a prairie chicken) did what prairie chickens did. He scratched in the dirt for seeds and insects. He clucked and cackled. And he flew in a thrashing of wings and feathers no more than a few feet off the ground. Why? Because that's how prairie chickens were supposed to fly.
>
> Years passed. One day he saw a magnificent bird soaring in the heavens with scarcely a beat of its strong golden wings. "What is the beautiful bird?" asked the eagle to his prairie chicken neighbor. "Why that's an eagle—the chief of all the birds," the neighbor replied. "But don't give it a second thought. You could never be like him."
>
> So the eagle never gave it a second thought. And thus he lived and died thinking he was a…prairie chicken.

One of the messages of the biblical book of Ecclesiastes is that many of us live like prairie chickens when we could soar like eagles. As a result, we scratch around in the dirt for life's meaning and never find it. "Vanity of vanities," cried the author of Ecclesiastes. I guess so. As long as we follow the crowd we'll end up just like them. At some point we must lift up our eyes and proclaim, "Enough!"—and break free.

God never planned for you to become submerged in the slimy swamp of the status quo. That doesn't mean that with God at the center of your life that you will automatically possess professional success, live free from financial concerns, or be completely healthy as long as you live. The gospel of health and wealth feels very empty to the faithful believer who struggles with sad circumstances not of his own choosing. The Job and Joseph stories of Scripture do a number on the automatic gospel of health and wealth that is often preached today. That's *not* what I'm talking about.

What I *am* talking about is this: You *can* take proactive steps to counteract the gravity pull of continued discouragement and defeat. After all, aren't you tired of living in the brown rut of mediocrity where every day is another shovelful of sameness? Aren't you tired of digging that same depressing ditch along with everyone else? Look up! Stretch your wings and soar like the eagle you were created to be.

On a cloudless and cool September afternoon, I stood on the back deck of a rental house overlooking the North Entrance to Yellowstone National Park over a mile away. A thousand feet below my perch was the wild and rushing Yellowstone River. With a panorama of mountains and valleys showcasing the colors of changing seasons, the most majestic sight of all was a lone bird that circled above. It was an eagle. If you have ever stopped and fixated your attention on God's magnificent creature you will appreciate the observation of Solomon who talked of things "too wonderful for me." And first on the wise man's list was "the way of an eagle in the sky" (Proverbs 30:18-19a). It's true. No one looks at an eagle in flight and says, "Oh, it's just another bird." There is no such thing as an eagle being *just another bird*. The soaring king of the heavens represents unintimidated courage, strong confidence, and invincible determination to be different from the majority. The fact is; no one thinks of the word "mediocrity" and eagle simultaneously. The eagle stands representatively as the very antithesis of managed average. So the haunting question you must answer is this: will you live your life like a prairie chicken scratching in the dirt like everyone else, or will you spread your wings and soar like the eagle God created you to be?

Food Fads and Pity Parties

I'm not sure why we make this health-thing so complicated. It's not. It really boils down to three non-negotiable essentials: (1) Drink water, (2) Eat real food, and (3) Exercise. We could possibly throw a fourth into the mix: Sleep. However, I've noticed that when I engage in the first three, rest usually comes easy.

We make it complicated with over-the-counter advice from a myriad of "experts" leaving our brains feeling like a closet full of clutter. In fact, we are surrounded by information overload to the point that we give up and conclude that living healthy is something beyond the scope of what normal people can do. It's exactly why diet-fad chasers burn out. There is always another "diet" on the market showcased by glamorous celebrities or beautiful models who guarantee weight loss and healthier living in "a few short weeks." *Really?* Such caters to the American quest for the quick fix. After all, we have fast-food, microwave meals, and drive-thru everything. Certainly on the day I decide to get healthy, there has to be something quick, fast, and easy. As Andrew (chapter one) said to me, "Too many people look for the easy way out. We have to be smarter than that." Indeed.

Speaking of smart, have you ever tried any of these "diets?"

- The Grapefruit Diet (sometimes called the Hollywood Diet)
- The Cambridge Diet
- Slim-Fast
- Lean Cuisine
- The South Beach Diet
- The Atkins Diet
- Weight Watchers
- Jenny Craig
- Nutri-System

That's not to say that certain elements of each of these did not and does not have their benefits. It is to say that many simply jump from one to another. As one lady said, "Dieting is the most active sport I have ever engaged in." Another admitted, "I yo-yo dieted myself to 250 pounds!"

Is it any wonder that while the food corporate giants are a billion-dollar industry, so is the weight-loss-diet industry? One literally "feeds" the other.

Listen to Julie...

I think I've lost two whole people with all the "diets" I pursued. Why is keeping it off so difficult? I loved buying those new clothes. No longer did I hesitate looking at myself in one of those mirrors at the clothing store. It was nice not going to the "Women's" side to look for something that made it look like it didn't come from "that" side of the store.

Yo-yo diets do more than destroy your confidence, they trick your body into thinking you can live one way only to realize within six months that the food is just like it used to be...fake. Here I am at age fifty-five and finally figured out what it takes to keep the weight off. I have been a master at knowing how to take it off and quite successful in putting it back on. But this time...it is different.

First, honesty within my family has lifted a heavy load. I haven't lied to my family; I just never shared this deep part of my soul. It is that painful. Weight loss journeys require openness with everyone and not just the trainer, the doctor, or the person at the weigh-in meeting. It begins with the people with whom you live; the people who see you day after day; the people who eat with you; the people who love you.

Second, I have to THINK about my choices. Here was my pattern: I lost weight and felt great. I bought new clothes. I looked better. So, I could now enjoy, eat what I wanted and do what others around me did. Never again would it appear like I was "dieting" because my plate could now look like yours. Wrong! Here's the deal I had to learn: I don't need to be like everyone else. I need to take care of me and do what I know is best for me. No one else can do it for me. I must THINK and make the decision daily to either destroy myself or lift myself up to health.

Third, healthy choices equal healthy lifestyles. This is not a "one and done" issue. Yes, you can lose weight and become a new you, but it's not over. You have to want to live healthy every day. We hear a lot about moderation. How do you get that? You get that through thinking about it. When I look at a menu, when I have an emotional moment, when I eat at someone's home, I have to

THINK about it. Do I have a small bite of this "forbidden" food, politely say, "No thank you" or just dive right in? And let me tell you that how you feel after you've made the decision will be your gauge as to whether or not you have accomplished moderation. Empower yourself! Take charge of you!

I wonder how many others found these diets to be quick-fix solutions that worked for a while but failed to address significant lifestyle changes. By the way, I once saw Slim-Fast spokesman and former Los Angeles Dodger baseball manager Tommy LaSorda at a Nashville area Cracker Barrel. We spoke for a moment during which I noticed he wasn't having Slim-Fast at all—but Tennessee biscuits and southern sausage gravy. So much for a Slim-Fast shake.

Regardless of advertising claims to the contrary, there is no quick and easy. It doesn't exist. If you want to get serious about your health, then *you* must get serious about your health. You don't eat right and exercise by proxy.

Question: Did you get out of shape and unhealthy overnight? No. My guess is, like most, you made bad choices that accumulated over time until the day you looked in the mirror and failed to recognize the person looking back. The only way to reverse the process is to reverse your thinking and decision making until healthy living becomes the habit of your lifestyle. And when you develop a healthy lifestyle, you will find the path to health, happiness, and wholeness.

One blogger who chronicles her weight loss journey (at 300+ pounds, she has a serious health situation) writes about her struggle while focusing on small steps of progress. After reading her early blogs, I'm not sure what steps she thinks she is taking. One day she asks, "Do you really expect me to go to a potluck with people from church that have made all this wonderful food and take my own salad and grilled chicken?" Uh, yes—if that's what it takes. On another day she writes what amounts to a personal congratulatory note and boasts that she has had fast-food only twice that week. Could that be twice too many? And yet another message confesses her comfort with a Snickers bar at one o'clock in the morning while sitting in front of her computer screen sending out her blog about her weight loss journey. If it is possible to be both blunt and kind then I'll be "kind" of "blunt"—if you are sitting in front of your computer at one o'clock in the morning with a Snickers candy bar, your weight loss journey will be non-existent.

Sorry, but drastic situations call for a drastic and immediate response.

At the risk of oversimplification, let's engage in an experiment. What if… we took away our blogger's "food addiction" and replaced it with "alcohol addiction"—what would your counsel be then? In fact, let's reword it to fit our substitution. (1) Do you really expect me to drive past this bar with all these friendly people and wonderful drinks and not partake? (2) I am making small steps of progress—I've only been drinking twice this week! (3) I'm sitting in front of my computer screen writing my blog about overcoming my drinking problem with a beer in my hand. Are you serious? Apparently not.

For an alcoholic to be successful with his/her turning point there must be a clear-cut decision, accountability, and a path for ridding himself/herself of all temptation. And it's the same with overeating. The crack addict has to go in search of a fix to feed his addiction. The food addict can find his on every corner under the dollar menu.

We do no one any favors by throwing pity parties and showering them with sympathy. (If you're looking for sympathy, you picked up the wrong book). An addict is exactly that. And until someone is willing to own it, become accountable, and make lifestyle changes, they will continue down the same yo-yo diet rut routine of losing fifteen pounds and gaining back twenty. Truth be known, there is no such thing as a successful "diet." The word "diet" is intended to be a noun, not a verb. In other words, weight loss and healthy living only happens when there is a long-term commitment to real lifestyle change.

There Is No Magic Pill

My Houston friend and physician, Ron Kirkwood, sums it up this way: "It's difficult to get patients to understand how much their weight is contributing to their poor health. Uncontrolled diabetes, elevated blood pressure from hypertension, painful joints, and increased risk from cardiac disease can all be attributed to their excessive weight. I offer this simple illustration. Suppose we are fishing in a boat on the lake when we hit a stump that punctures the bottom of the boat. We would use buckets and whatever else we can find to bail water in order to safely reach the shore. However, before we take the boat back out again, we would need to fix the hole. Prescribing medication is analogous to my handing them another bucket to keep afloat. What they really need is to repair the boat i.e., repair themselves by losing the weight."

He's right. Sadly the American M.O. is to see an M.D. for the magic pill. And if he won't give us one, we'll find another doctor who will.

Since overweight people now represent the majority of Americans, it's time for physicians to close the door, take a deep breath, look their patients in the eye, and tell the truth. It may not be what we *want* to hear, but it is definitely what we *need* to hear. We need more physicians who will stop trying to be politically and socially correct and who will get specific with their patients about their food choices and needed lifestyle changes. We need to be told with a sit-down-look-in-the-eye bluntness that certain eating habits and a lack of exercise are killing us and…setting up our children for a lifestyle of disease and early death. Many times it takes a doctor—who cares about us enough to communicate this unpleasant truth—before we will listen.

An Apple a Day Keeps the Doctor Away

My Mom said that and my guess is that your Mom did, too. When God created fruits and vegetables, He loaded them up with all the essential things needed to build a healthy immune system. In other words, one of the best ways to practice prevention (keep from getting sick) is to understand the importance of good nutrition. And that's where God's garden variety of fruits and vegetables come in.

For one thing, fruits and vegetables provide antioxidants needed for healthy cells. And we have a lot of cells. Those cells are our body's front-line defense against oxidative stress. What does that mean? It means that our cells tend to break down (causing premature aging and disease) unless they are buoyed by antioxidants. And where do I get antioxidants? A bag of Cheetos? A fistful of M&M's? A pint of Haagen Daz? Uh, no. This is where you hear the drum roll...*fruits and vegetables!*

Take an apple, for example. Did you know there are over 10,000 nutrients in a single apple? 10,000? Yes. You have a little bit of everything packed into a single apple. And all of these ingredients work together as a team to protect your body from sickness. While science and a study of nutrition was never my thing; what *is* my thing is living better and healthier. Studies have proven that eating a diet rich in fruits and vegetables actually decrease the risk for heart disease. So, how do I get all the good stuff in an apple? How about this: eat one. And tomorrow eat another one. Maybe that's why Bob Harper's *Skinny Rules* lists this as Rule #6: "Eat Apples and Berries Every Single Day—EVERY SINGLE DAY!" Our moms were right.

The flip side is that it's just as easy not to eat an apple a day. Carter Hays echoes the same in his book, *Discover Your Road to Divine Health*, "The difference [in eating or not eating an apple a day] is that you choose *to*, or *not* to. I don't mean to be too simplistic or seem uncaring, but it really is that simple." Each day we are faced with a series of choices—eat better/ live better or eat worse/get sick (and sicker). Either way you will pay the price. You either pay up front for wellness or pay on the back end for sickness. Here's a "duh" question: Which do you think will eventually cost you more?

Supersize Me

In the 2004 documentary film, *Supersize Me*, Morgan Spurlock takes a firsthand look at America's obesity crisis by chronicling his own physical journey over a thirty-day period in which he ate only McDonald's food. He ate at the popular fast food restaurant three times each day and tried everything on their menu at least once. When employees asked if he wanted his meal "Supersized," he said yes. A typical meal consisted of a Double Quarter Pounder with cheese, super sized French fries, and a 42-ounce Coke. He gained 9.5 pounds in just the first five days. By the end of thirty days, he had gained 24.5 pounds. Physicians were surprised at the rapid deterioration of his health.

The fast food giant fought back claiming Spurlock's 5,000 calorie per day diet did not include any exercise and that such would have happened regardless of where he ate. Still other reviewers stated that regardless of the unscientific nature of the study, the overall message was clear: fast food is not good for you.

There is a simple reason why we are getting bigger—it's cheap and easy. Americans are now eating out as much (if not more) than they are eating at home, restaurant portions are twice as large as they were a few years ago, fast food (filled with salt, sugar, and fat) tastes good, and many "value meals" come with standard high calorie sodas included. Popular comedian Tim Hawkins does a spoof on a movie theater concessions operator who charges $8 for a 44 ounce soft drink who then says in surfer-dude-speak: "…And for twenty-five cents more, man, you can get a 64-ounce soft drink with free refills." Hawkins adds, "Hey, if you're drinking 64 ounces of soft drink and need a refill, MAN, YOU'VE GOT A PROBLEM!"

It's essential we get to the place where large colas and supersized fries are not only not tempting to us, but actually repulsive (or at least seen as a once-in-a-while special treat). Hey, no one said lifestyle change comes easy. The easiest thing is to continue to give in and go along, but that doesn't seem to be working very well.

By the way, you can't outrun a Big Mac Value Meal! McDonald's staple sandwich alone is 540 calories. Add a large fry and a soft drink and you are up to whopping 1,350 in total calories (speaking of "whopping"—a Burger King Whopper value meal is 1,430 calories). Compare that to an hour-long four-mile walk which burns an average of 350 calories. I'm not good at math, but subtracting the former from the latter leaves one in the calorie red. In other words, you would have to walk approximately four hours to break even. When you realize how hard it is to "work off" a Big Mac "Value Meal," you may want to re-think your choices (unless you want to put up some Forest Gump type numbers and run all the way to Malibu!). "Value Meals" are not very valuable.

Every study I've read from the "experts" say the same thing. You must eat to lose. It sounds like a contradiction until you understand that what they are saying is this: **you must eat the right food—real food—in order**

to lose. As *Biggest Loser* trainer Bob Harper says, "You've got to get the engine going for the engine to use all the extra fuel that's hanging around your waist." Soda, candy, and chips are not the right food. And neither is fast food fare loaded with salt, sugar, and fat. We need protein along with a "garden" variety of nutrient-rich foods in order to live well. To paraphrase the sentiments of nutritionists—*if there are ingredients on that food label you can't pronounce, keep walking!*

Debbi Anderson Patton Walton (certified personal trainer, specialist in post-rehab, and wellness coach in Huntsville, Alabama) asks,

> "What are you running on? Every machine is designed to run on a specific kind of fuel. For example, if you fill your car with a lower octane gas than it was designed to use, you will experience less power (energy) and worse performance. If you continue to use the cheaper fuel, your engine will eventually suffer damage. It's the same with the most amazing machine of all—your body.
>
> Your body was designed to run mostly on plants. The more quantity and variety, the more energy and protection you will give your body. The thousands of phytochemicals (or phytonutrients) found in a wide variety of plants, fuel your energy, protect you from disease, and help you maintain your youth, vigor, and vitality. This is non-negotiable. Without a wide variety of fruits and vegetables in your diet, it's not if you get sick; it's when and how sick will you be? You choose every day what you put in your mouth. Do you prefer sluggish, dragging, depressed, or high gear optimal peak performance? To a great extent you choose your health and performance by choosing your fuel. So, upon what kind of fuel are you running?"

Carter Hays injects a touch of humor when he says, "Since an apple is real food, your body knows what to do with it. On the other hand, your body is completely confused by a bag of Doritos. *What do I do with this?*—it asks. And because your body doesn't know what to do with it, it decides to simply store it until it can figure it out. So, it stores it—*around your waist!*"

It is estimated that the fast food industry spends in excess of $4 billion annually advertising its salt, sugar, and fat offerings—much of which is aimed at kids. As Mika Brzezinski reports, "By comparison, for every dollar the industry spends pushing fast food, the U.S. Department of Agriculture spends about one-tenth of a penny encouraging people to eat their vegetables." That's hardly a level playing field. Then, again, parents must do a better job stepping up and leading by example. Grocery stores do the same thing by placing candy and sugary snacks strategically where children can see them. Once more, parents must *parent*. Someone has to be the adult in the room (or aisle).

The Family Table

My grandmother's full time job seemed to be gardening and cooking. And although my mother taught high school, she seemed to spend a lot of time meal-planning and cooking. Growing up in the 1960s our family table was a special place. We seldom ate out in those days (we couldn't afford it) and when we did it was a treat. We began our mornings at the family table with breakfast and ended it at the same place for supper (I think more well-to-do families called it "dinner," but it was always "supper" at our house). It was a time we shared more than a home-cooked meal. We shared the day's anticipations as well as its realities. We told stories. We laughed. We had fun. We acted silly. We were a family and we ate together. When television came along and TV trays were the rage, my dad gave in—but *only* on Saturday nights. I have no idea what was on television those nights, but I do remember the excitement of eating on those plastic trays.

Fast forward fifty years and today "made from scratch" seems to be a hobby reserved for the Amish. Food is microwavable, pre-packaged and processed where it is poured easily from a box or a can. And the idea of eating together as a family has all but disappeared from the American landscape. We eat on the run and seldom give much thought as to what exactly we're eating. As long as it tastes good (as in salt, sugar, and fat), we're good to go (literally). Physician David Katz says, "Everything about modern living that makes it modern is obesigenic. The problem is a flood of highly processed, hyperpalatable, energy-dense, nutrient-diluted, glow-in-the-dark, bet-you-can't eat-just-one kind of foods." It's been called "the perfect storm" of overeating.

Yet in a measured defense of family life in our times, I must say that as a father of four there were days when we did the best we could. Between baseball, football, soccer practices, school functions, church services, and dozens of other activities vying for our time, there were some evenings when we grabbed a burger from the Little League concession stand or found supper in a sack via the drive-thru at Wendy's. Nothing I am suggesting here is over-the-top idealistic (or unrealistic). Sometimes it is what it is. Been there. Done that. Enough said.

Sadly, however, that is all some families ever know.

One of the best tools to avoid obesity and help your kids make better and healthier choices is eating together as a family whenever possible. Multiple studies have shown the benefits—families who eat several meals per week at the family table have kids who make better grades and have a lesser tendency toward drug abuse. Studies aside, common sense should tell you the same. Besides, it's also a great time to teach table manners, talk about life-stuff, and foster better communication. It may have been one of the principles behind Moses' counsel to young parents in Deuteronomy 6—"You shall teach them diligently to your sons and shall talk of them when you sit in your house and when you walk by the way and when you lie down and when you rise up" (verse 7). So, pull your kids away from the TV, laptop, and iPhone (anything that plugs in) and pull them up to the table. Rediscovering the benefits of family meal time will pay multiple dividends.

Are we living longer? Yes.

Are we living better? It's a good question. What answer would you give?

CHAPTER 4

Betcha Can't Eat Just One!

At mealtime Boaz said to her, "Come here, that you may eat of the
bread and dip your piece of bread in the vinegar." So she sat beside
the reapers; and he served her roasted grain, and she ate and was
satisfied and had some left. (Ruth 2:14)

The huge processed food manufacturers know exactly what they are
doing—Pillsbury, Post, Nestle, Kraft, General Foods (both Kraft and
General Foods are owned by Phillip Morris, the huge tobacco company),
General Mills, Proctor and Gamble, Frito-Lay, Coca-Cola, Kellogg, and
dozens more—are experts in knowing what we crave and giving it to us
in ways that maximize taste, convenience, and cost. They know how to
package, promote, and give their foods the pizzazz needed to go flying
off of grocer's shelves. The food giants have dominated the American diet,
reshaped the way we eat, and made untold millions in the process.

There are three pillars of processed foods that have played a major role
in the obesity crisis: salt, sugar, and fat. Salt jolts the taste buds the very
moment we tear off the shinny wrapper and take the first bite. Sugar,
according to studies, lights up the brain in much the same was as does
cocaine. Fat delivers its loads of calories and leaves us literally hungering
for more. In recent years as consumers grew more health conscious by
demanding more healthy choices, the food giants responded favorably.
Well, sort of. According to Michael Moss (*Salt, Sugar, Fat—How the Food
Giants Hooked Us*), the food industry's most devious ploy thus far and the

one they wish to keep secret is this—"lowering one bad boy ingredient like fat while quietly adding more sugar to keep people hooked."

It's a marketing home run (in fact, it's a grand slam!). They have successfully retooled their packaging by offering "Low-Fat" "Lot-Sodium" "Reduced Sugar" alternatives that grab the headlines of the box or bottle and thus attract health-conscious consumers like the mom who wants the best for her kids. However, rather than place a product on the shelf that now tastes like cardboard, they reduce one "gotcha" ingredient only to maximize another. In other words, they do whatever it takes to keep the taste in tact. And we buy it. Literally.

In some cases, they merely change the name. Remember Sugar Crisp, Sugar Smacks, and Sugar Frosted Flakes? The breakfast moguls didn't change the ingredients—only the names. Thus they are marketed today as more healthy breakfast choices under the redesigned logo of Super Golden Crisp, Honey Smacks, and Frosted Flakes. Gone is the word "sugar" from the front of the box. Of course, it's still in the cereal (and in incredible amounts), but you'll only read it in the finer print on the side of the box. They are betting on the fact that you won't notice. And most don't.

Remember the old saying, "Fool me once, shame on you. Fool me twice, shame on me." Indeed, it's shame on me.

It is imperative that we educate ourselves and become smarter when it comes to the creations of crave. There are three ingredients that food producers use in massive quantities to create the perfect storm of unhealthy eating, get us hooked, and keep us coming back for more.

The Perfect Storm: Sugar

It had already been a long day and made even longer by my teaching a Wednesday night class at church. Our son, Luke, was home with a sore throat and, per his request; we stopped by our neighborhood supermarket to pick up some Italian Ice. Handing him the small six-ounce container of the lemon-flavored ice only reminded me of how good it tastes. I grabbed one for myself. Finishing it quickly, I took a second. I mean, how bad could a meager six ounces be (okay, twelve ounces)? I read the ingredients and *WHOA!* It contained 20 grams of sugar *per serving*. Let's see, twenty grams of sugar calculates to approximately five teaspoons of sugar (one teaspoon of granulated white sugar equals 4.2 grams). And I had eaten two of those things. No wonder it tasted good! It was nothing more than ice-cotton candy melting in my mouth. Yum!

God supplied us with some ten thousand taste buds to differentiate various flavors. Those taste buds go crazy when sugar is present by sending instantaneous messages to the brain that this is really, really, *really* good. We are, after all, hard-wired for sweet. And manufacturers know it all too well. Truth be known, the average American consumes 22 teaspoons of sugar per day. To understand the concept in even more familiar terms, consider that to be the same as eating 22 sugar cubes per day. Additionally, we drink approximately 30-40 gallons of sugar soft drinks per person per year. And when you add sweetened teas, sport drinks and vitamin water, it bumps up to an additional 14 gallons per person per year. All told, that's a lot of mouth-watering sweet stuff. Sugar's effect on our brains is so strong that scientists view certain sugary foods as potentially addictive.

Sugar has no equal when it comes to creating crave and no one consumes more of it per person that the residents of the United States. And while there has been a decrease in physical exercise over the past three decades, no one attributes America's obesity epidemic to the mere reduction in physical activity. There's more to it than that. And *it* is called…"sugar."

By the way, even the sweetness of smell bombards the brain's pleasure zones. If you don't believe that, walk around the cocoa plant in Chocolate-Town, USA (Hershey, Pennsylvania). Without discipline, the smell will send you straight to their chocolate store (which is probably what they want you to do).

The American Heart Association has gone on record to connect the excessive consumption of sugar to the pandemic of obesity and cardiovascular disease. Noting that the average American was consuming 22 teaspoons per day, the AHA recommended our sugar intake be reduced to a more healthy 5 teaspoons for women and 9 teaspoons for men. And what did the food industry do about the AHA warnings? They did the same as the rest of us—not much at all.

Sugar dominates most of our food products. It's why Campbell's Prego

(Italian for "you're welcome") brand of spaghetti sauce is so good. The largest ingredient (after tomatoes) is...sugar. One half cup of Prego Traditional sauce has as much sugar as three Oreo cookies. As they say in Italy, "Mama-mia!" *You're welcome!*

We start our mornings with sugar. When John Glenn orbited the earth for NASA in 1962, he came home touting the wonder drink "Tang." Sales "rocketed" just like the astronaut. Tang was nothing more than chemicals and sugar. While Pop Tarts contain a hint of fruit, they also contain 19 grams of sugar (more than four teaspoons). Do we really want our kids consuming "Chocolate Chip Cookie Dough Pop-Tarts" for breakfast? A glass of sugar Tang and a Pop Tart... And we wonder why kids have health/obesity/behavioral issues?

The problem is, we seek to balance convenience with healthy eating. That's exactly why Betty Crocker became one of the most famous women in America in the 1960s. She preached convenience and quickly developed a fan base that rivaled athletes and rock stars. It is said she received over a thousand fan letters per day. The irony was that Betty Crocker never existed—a mere figment of the advertising imagination by the folks at General Mills. However, she transformed the American kitchen into the "shake and bake," "heat and serve" it is today and was thus heralded by millions of moms nationwide. Who is concerned about ingredients when you can serve it fast, quick, and easy? Thus convenience became the fourth tenet of the revised American Declaration of Independence which now promises "life, liberty, the pursuit of happiness"—and *convenience.*

And when it comes to cereal—the staple of the American breakfast—investigative reporter, Michael Moss (*Salt, Sugar, Fat—How the Food Giants Hooked Us*) asked the pertinent question: "Is it cereal or is it candy?" Good question. With more and more women in the workforce and rushing out the door next to their children, breakfast became a source of stress. Once again, convenience won the day.

It's no secret that the big three breakfast giants (General Mills, Post, and Kellogg) aim their marketing strategies at kids. When America's children were glued to the television for Saturday morning cartoons, the sweetest cereal brands were advertised. Given catchy cartoon characters like Tony the Tiger ("They're G-r-r-r-eat!), what kid wouldn't grab for the nearest box of Frosted Flakes, Count Chocula, Captain Crunch, or Sugar Smacks? In other words, sugar in a box. When the public began to wise up about sugar, the box labels were changed to protect the innocent (the processed food companies). Sugar content remained about the same. Even fruit sounding titles were/are misleading. The largest ingredient, for example, in Apple Jacks isn't apples—it's sugar (13.7 grams).

At this point I owe my wonderful sister-in-law an apology. Joanie always had an eye toward healthy eating. My brother, however, looked forward to my visits because it gave him the excuse he needed to head to the grocery store where he would rummage happily through the cereal isle in search of his beloved Cocoa Krispies—his cereal of choice and one banned from their home. But since I was visiting and company came first, he bought, he ate, and I received the blame.

Like two unruly adolescents, we ate junk, laughed, and slurped our way back to the sugary bliss of childhood. So, here goes...

Dear Joanie:

My dear sister-in-law, I am so sorry. Please accept my humble apology for corrupting your dear husband. I'm not sure what our penance should be, but on my next visit you can take us to the store and purchase the cereal of *your* choice—and then watch us eat it.

And then there are the cola wars.

The cola wars make the cereal wars look like child's play. Coca-Cola is the most powerful brand name in the world. As the beverage maker's profits soared, so did America's waistline. Ask any nutritionist or fitness expert about the value of soft drinks and they will immediately scowl. Nothing is considered more to be the root cause behind obesity than soda. Mika Brzezinski (*Obsessed*) writes, "As far as I am concerned, if you wipe all soda off the face of the earth, this would be a better place. I don't know any reason why anyone should serve soda to their kids. It's like letting them drink candy. It's nothing more than liquid sugar..." Medical experts suggest sugary drinks to be suspect number one in the diabetes epidemic. Bob Harper says about contestants on *The Biggest Loser,* "When I reviewed their pre-*TBL* meal plans, I saw that most contestants were drinking Big Gulps or other massive jugs of soda..." He goes on to say that some drank as many as 1,500 calories of soda a day!

"The main thing is excess calories," according to Dr. Christopher Ochner, assistant professor of pediatrics and adolescent medicine at the Icahn School of Medicine at Mount Sinai. In an interview with FoxNews.com, Dr. Ochner went on to add, "If everything else in their diet is equal, a person who has a can of Coke a day, adds an extra 14.5 pounds per year, just for the calories alone." One can of Coke per day doesn't sound like much. However, 14.5 pounds sounds like much. If you don't think so, pick up fifteen or so pounds and carry that around for a while. Not only does it "weigh" you down, but it hangs around—your waist! Think of calories as dessert. Why would anyone drink dessert? We must become smarter than that.

Once more, the issue isn't the occasional 12-ounce can of Coke. The issue has become the American drive to *supersize!* That's why the soft drink companies were eager to replace the 12-ounce cans (9 teaspoons of sugar) with 20-ounce bottles (15 teaspoons of sugar) that dot the nation's coolers and vending machine landscape. Just to place some perspective...

12 ounce can of Coke = 39 grams of sugar (9 teaspoons)

20 ounce bottle of Coke = 65 grams of sugar (15 teaspoons)

1 liter bottle of Coke = 108 grams of sugar (26 teaspoons)

44 ounce Super Big Gulp of Coke = 128 grams of sugar (30 teaspoons)

64 ounce Double Gulp of Coke = 186 grams of sugar (44 teaspoons)

If you translated each of those teaspoons into simple sugar cubes, what parent in their right mind would hand their kids nine cubes of sugar to eat—much less 44? And yet, the average American kid drinks 20 ounces of liquid candy per day. And "average" means that many are consuming much more.

It's no accident that the beverage companies who own the drink territory in fast food restaurants want their brand bundled with a "value meal" and where you service yourself at the all-you-can-drink beverage bar. They simply sell more that way. And what is the key ingredient driving our craving for more? Sugar.

In 1980, soft drink manufacturers switched from typical table sugar to the less expensive fructose-corn syrup. As Bob Harper asks, "When factory farms want to fatten their cattle, what do they do? They feed them corn. So if you are drinking things with corn syrup, think about that. Are you a cow? No, you are not." And even as soft drink consumption slips as the public becomes more health conscious, the rise in sweetened teas, sports drinks, and sugar water has increased.

It's no secret that soda is one of the top sellers in the grocery industry. From end-of-the-aisle eye-catching displays to the checkout zone where twenty ounce bottles are lined up next to the register and readily available to the impulse buyer (beverage distributers and store owners know that the majority of grocery purchases are unplanned), Coke is king. In fact, Coke is like the giant Xerox, in that "Coke" is the southern generic term for all soft drinks (much to the chagrin of Pepsi).

One additional ploy has been fostered upon the gullible public by the food corporations: fruit. By adding a tablespoon of fruit juice, non-carbonated sugary drinks are now packaged and sold as a healthy fruit drink. After all, given the choice between a cola and Kool-Aid, the picture of fruit on the packaging can make all the difference. As Moss' research showed, "Some of Capri Sun's [fruit drink marketed by General Foods] flavors were higher in sugar than soda." Yet they find themselves packed into the lunch sacks of America's kids every school day. And why not? Their packages are covered with pictures of...*fruit*.

I picked up a carton of juice last week covered in pictures of lemons, cherries, oranges, and bananas. I read the small print: "Contains No Fruit Juice." Amazing! It did contain a boatload of sugar.

Are we hooked on sugar? You decide. By the way, the jury is still out on the "diet" drinks. Studies show that even the "diet" colas filled with artificial sweeteners only serve to whet the appetite for more sweets.

Wise up, America! If you want fruit—eat *fruit*. If you want a drink—drink *water* (or unsweet teas or black coffee). And read the labels. They are there for a reason. Ignore them and it may be you or someone you love receiving the dreaded diagnosis of...diabetes.

The Perfect Storm: Fat

Fat and sugar combined are the dynamic duo of food synergy. Food consumption depends upon one thing only: *taste*. If food tastes good, we eat it. If we eat it, we buy more of it. On the other hand, if it tastes like cardboard, we spit it out and move on. Food companies producing non-fatty cardboard are soon out of business.

Fat is what throws the party in our mouths. It puts the crunch into potato chips, the crisp into fried chicken, and adds the creamy smooth mouth-feel to our ice cream. In fact, what happens in our mouths is similar to the burgers on the backyard grill dripping with fat and surrounded by the exploding flames. Fat is finger-lickin' good and the food companies know it.

There is only one problem (well, more than one, but we'll go with one). Fat has a terrible public relations image. Sugar, on the other hand (at least until America became smarter) has had a positive image. It conjures up pictures of everything that is sweet and good. After all American grandmothers love to pinch the cheeks of grandbabies while asking for a little "sugar." Southern gentlemen often refer to their sweetheart (there's that "sweet" again) as "Shug" (short for "sugar"). Even salt has long been viewed as favorable. Most men of the post-WWII generation wanted it on the table and used it generously. Even the Bible compares Christ-followers to "the salt of the earth" (Matthew 5:13).

Not so with fat. Fat in foods is usually connected with fat on the body. Studies show that the first ingredient shoppers look for when they read labels is fat content. As a result, "Low-Fat" and "Fat-Free" items have flooded store shelves leaving consumers feeling better and healthier about their choices (and, as previously noted, tricked by crafty marketing). However, not all fats are bad. Good fats are found in the foods God made and man hasn't messed with (avocado, raw nuts, real butter, eggs, fatty fish and whole milk).

Take milk. In an effort to be health-conscious, my parents passed on the whole milk and bought 2%. And why not—if 98% of the fat has been removed (which is what most people think that means). But that's not what that means. The truth is; the fat content of whole milk is only 3% anyway. So, we paid more money and got a fat savings of a grand total of…1%.

Today our family drinks skim milk because we are concerned about the fat. Of course, like so many American families, we more than make up for it with fat-filled cheese. In fact, cheese has become the single largest source of saturated fat in our diets to the tune of 33 pounds of cheese per person per year—up from 11 pounds in 1970. At the same time, milk went from 25 gallons per person per year in 1970 to about six gallons today. We simply traded milk for cheese. And in a very big way.

Remember those Chef Boyardee pizzas your mom used to make? They weren't exactly loaded with cheese. So, fast forward to the frozen pizzas of today that advertize "Triple Cheese" or "Cheese Baked into the Crust!" Cheese is the reason frozen DiGiorno pizza sales have reaped hefty rewards for the parent company, Kraft. We have cheese on our breakfast sandwiches, cheese on our lunch sandwiches, cheese added to our baked potato, smothering our enchiladas, or melted onto our chicken breast at Applebee's. We love fatty cheese. Of course, we wouldn't dare drink milk that's not "skim." Got to watch the fat, you know. We are so inconsistently funny.

Then again, what would happen if food companies gave us low-fat cheese? No one would eat it. It's all about taste.

Fat is what makes ice cream **taste** so good. Fat is what makes pizza **taste** so good. Fat is what makes anything fried **taste** so good. The problem *isn't* that we take the grandkids to eat ice cream for an occasional treat, eat pizza with friends on Sunday night, or enjoy a fish fry. The problem *is* that we do it too often and consume enormous portions.

And fat sells. The average American mom has three "C's" in mind when shopping for her family: (1) cost, (2) kids, (3) convenience. (Okay, make that two "C's" and 1 "K.") In other words, is it cheap, will my kids eat it, and is it quick? Fat answers those three questions with a resounding "Yes!" "Yes!" and "Yes!"

In March, 2008, I surprised my wife with a 50th birthday getaway trip to Savannah, Georgia. The azaleas were in full bloom and the city parks were alive with the spark of southern spring. Savannah is a beautiful city with the perfect combination of old south meets young eclectic. It's also the home of Julie's favorite cook: Paula Deen. We enjoyed dining in her famous The Lady and Sons restaurant where we soaked up both southern charm and southern cooking at its finest.

Paula Deen isn't exactly the queen of healthy cuisine. In fact, it was rare on her cooking show when she made anything that wasn't loaded with saturated fat (whole sticks of butter were her trademarks) while licking her fingers and saying in her sweet southern drawl, "This is good, y'all!"

Kraft was watching, too. They hired her to ramp up their slugging Philadelphia Cream Cheese brand. Paula Deen used social media to promote a contest in which Kraft offered $25,000 to the winners who submitted the best recipe via YouTube using their famous cream cheese. My wife couldn't hit the kitchen fast enough. She came up with a recipe; we filmed it, placed it on YouTube and waited for the phone to ring. It didn't ring. Little did we know that the Kraft Corporation was inundated with thousands of Paula Deen fans all doing the same thing. Sales of Philadelphia Cream Cheese took off.

Sadly in 2012, Deen announced that she had been diagnosed with diabetes as early as 2009. Her fans were stunned. The fat-filled food for which she was known had actually paved the way for her illness. In her defense, she insisted in interviews that she preached and practiced moderation. Regardless, like the queen of southern cooking herself, America was forced to re-evaluate her love affair with fatty foods.

The Perfect Storm: Salt

Sodium is an essential nutrient that keeps the body in balance. Of all the aspects of a healthy diet, however, the toughest one to achieve is keeping the sodium to a reasonable and recommended level.

Physicians like those associated with the Mayo Clinic recommend 2,300 milligrams as the optimum amount of sodium adults should consume daily. For those over fifty and anyone with diabetes, high blood pressure, or kidney disease, the number drops to 1,500 milligrams per day. Here's the health kicker (literally). Americans consume on average 3,800 mg of salt a day! Michael F. Jacobson, Ph.D. and Director, Center for Science in the Public Interest says, "That extra sodium may be the most dangerous thing in our diet, unnecessarily killing tens of thousands of people every year due to heart attacks and strokes" (*Nutrition Action*, July 2013). It has been called the leading cause of premature death.

It's not the salt shaker on the American kitchen table that is the culprit. It has been estimated that as much as 80% of our sodium intake comes from processed foods. Consider…

- The microwavable frozen roast turkey dinner from Hungry Man delivers 5,400 mg of salt—enough sodium for two days! –And that's if you don't eat anything else.

- The smoked turkey breast sandwich at Panera Bread contains 1,650 mg.

- The Lasagna Classico at Olive Garden has 2,830 mg.

- The three ounce package of Top Ramen Noodles in our pantry (a favorite of college students everywhere) has 910 mg. of sodium *per serving*. Seriously, who eats only half of the small package (one serving). Do the math. Eat the entire three ounces (which isn't much) and you are rewarded with 1820 mg of sodium. That's 80% of all the salt needed in one day!

- The Kikkoman Soy Sauce on the table at our favorite Chinese restaurant contains 920 mg of sodium per serving. I've seen people pour it liberally on their rice and food and undoubtedly getting twice and three times that amount. Come to think of it, *I* have poured it liberally on *my* rice and food.

- Campbell's V8 Vegetable Juice is supposed to be a healthy substitute for vegetables (FYI: there is no such thing as a healthy substitute for the real thing) but contains as much as 480 mg of sodium per serving. When consumer groups protested, they reduced the sodium level to 420 mg—*per serving*.

- An average cup of Campbell's regular Condensed Soup has 760 mg of sodium. In other words, liquid salt! Of course, most people consume the entire can. At 2.5 servings it totals to 1,900 mg of salt—enough salt intake for the entire day!

- A Nestlé Pepperoni and Three Cheese Calzone Hot Pocket contains 750 mg of sodium (and three teaspoons of sugar). Look closely again—

that's for only one half of the calzone. Do the math. No one eats half of a calzone.

- Marie Callender's Chicken Pot Pie has been a personal favorite for years. It has 520 calories and 800 mg of sodium. I might have "lived" with that until I happened to notice the package contains *two servings*. Are you kidding? Who eats only half a pot pie? Not me. So...one pie equates to 1,040 calories and 1,600 mg of sodium. Say it's not so, Marie.

- A single container of Healthy Choice Cheese Tortellini soup does better at 390 mg of sodium. But it's also for two servings. Yet even at 780 mg, our son wouldn't eat it. "It tastes terrible," he said.

Reduce sodium to reasonable levels that would fulfill the health requirement of 2,300 mg per day for the average healthy adult and...you produce food that tastes, well, terrible. When I ate a cup of Progresso Healthy Classic Vegetable Soup last week, it contained 466 mg of salt. It was all I could do to keep from reaching for the shaker. We have become so accustomed to salt. And the food folks know it.

Food manufacturers don't just add salt to our diets—they dump salt into our mac & cheese, spaghetti sauces, pizzas, and salad dressings. It's the salt that gives our food its taste appeal. It's why the movie popcorn is so appealing and why we eat every last bite of it. It's why we set out to eat only a handful of Cheez-It crackers or Lays Potato Chips and find that you really can't eat just one. As Michael Moss writes, "Without salt, processed food companies cease to exist."

The country of Finland knows this. Given the high incidence of cardiovascular disease in their country, the Finns took action. Like tobacco warnings on the side of cigarettes, they place the warning: "High Salt Content" on grocery items that exceed recommended levels. By 2007 Finland's per capita salt consumption was down by a third and deaths from heart attacks and strokes were down 80 percent. Is this a mere coincidence?

Salt, however, makes us feel good. The food that makes you feel good is the food you naturally want to buy—and more of it. And the food that makes you feel good is the food that tastes good. And the foods that taste good taste that way because they are loaded with sodium. By the way, we aren't born liking salt. While babies are born liking sugar, they will wrinkle up their cute little noses at salt. It's an acquired taste—and an addictive one.

Last Saturday I had two options when it came to syrup on Julie's waffles. There was Pure Maple Syrup (which listed one ingredient: Maple Syrup) or Aunt Jemima's Original Lite. The ingredients on the Aunt Jemima Lite bottle included high fructose corn syrup (that's a no-no), salt, sodium benzoate (a salt-preservative that prevents mold), and sodium hexametaphosphate (a really cool word to say, but it's really a water-softener) and several "artificial and natural flavors" which makes the syrup taste like...well, syrup. Hence, salt and/or sodium were mentioned three times. The bottle advertised "50% Fewer Calories" (what consumers want). The "fewer calories," however, comes with a catch: there is no maple syrup. There is, however, a bunch of chemicals along with high fructose corn syrup and...salt.

I love potato chips and all kinds. Given the choice between a piece of chocolate cake and a handful of chips, I'll go for the chips. Maybe it goes back to my elementary school days when we toured the potato chip factory. Maybe it's the crunch. My guess is...it's the salt.

Moss reports that the average American eats twelve pounds of those things each year. I know some who have switched from chips to pretzels (less fat). My guess is they don't know that pretzels have triple the sodium of potato chips (Cheetos have almost twice as much). It's little surprise that the *New England Journal of Medicine* published the report that every four years since 1986, we gain an average of 3.55 pounds. And what were the top contributors to our national weight gain? Red meat, sugar-sweet drinks, and potato chips—the staples of the American diet.

Read the label on a bag of chips. The serving size is usually measured at one ounce. Does anyone eat a mere one ounce? Come on... My guess is that it's not uncommon for consumers to *consume* the whole bag! And why not? Loaded with salt, sugar (carbohydrate), and fat, the potato chip provides the taste buds with instant gratification by sending messages of pleasure flying off to the brain that seek more of the same. They were right... *you can't eat just one.* Well, you can, but no one does.

Then there's fast (and salty) food. Keep in mind the recommended requirement for healthy adults under fifty is 2,300 mg per day. For everyone else it's 1,500. Here are ten salty goodies…

- Quiznos Large French Dip—a popular prime rib sandwich with all the trimmings and served with a side of au jus will add 3,610 mg of sodium (not to mention 1,200 calories). This sandwich might better be called "The Salt Bomb."

- Arby's fried mozzarella sticks (a count of six) have 2,530 mg of sodium—more than an entire days worth.

- McDonald's big breakfast with hot cakes comes in at 2,260 mg of sodium.

- Taco Bell's Volcano Nachos contain 1,670 mg of sodium (not to mention 58 grams of fat).

- Subway's Spicy Italian sandwich without sauces or cheese contains 1,520 mg. Make it a foot-long with mayo and you're up to 3,200 mg of sodium.

- Eat a KFC Variety Big Box Meal along with mashed potatoes and gravy, cole slaw, a biscuit and a 32-ounce Pepsi (standard lunch fare for many) and you will blast off with 3,000 mg of sodium.

- Papa John's Buffalo Chicken Pizza contains 1,050 per slice (which works only if you eat one slice).

- Hardee's 2/3-lb Monster Thickburger contains 1,300 calories, 93 grams of fat and…2,860 mg of sodium. That's doesn't count fries and a soda.

- A loaded-up Chipotle Burrito (ingredients may vary) can contain up to 2,650 mg of sodium. Surprise: the flour tortilla is the worst salt culprit with 670 mg alone.

- A McDonald's Big Mac Value Meal weighs in at 1,470 mg of sodium or over 60% of a recommended daily allowance.

And then there are all those sodium ingredients that you're not sure what they are—except more salt. Looking again at the small three ounce packaging for Top Ramen Oodles of Noodles it lists among its ingredients: salt, sodium carbonate, sodium tripolyphosphate, disodium guanylate, disodium inosinate, and sodium alginate. I'm no chemist, but I'm guessing that represents salt in different forms and...a lot of it.

Moss quotes from Robert I-San Lin, a chief scientist with Frito-Lay (Doritos, Cheetos, Fritos) from 1974 to 1982, whose job was to develop products that would keep consumers coming back for more. Looking back on his work years later, Moss reports Lin's feelings of regret. "I feel so sorry for the public," he said. FYI: *you* are the public for whom he feels sorry.

Where Does That Leave Us?

From the aisles of the grocery's stores to the drive thru of America's fast food favorites, it's easy to see why we are heavier, unhealthier, and spending untold amounts of money managing our sick care. Sadly and truthfully, Americans are hooked on supersized salty, sugary, fatty, and cheap foods that are making us sick and slowly killing us.

My wife and I were riding along today and discussing the contents of this chapter. "I feel duped," she said. So do I. So do a lot of people who figure it out.

You will never find your turning point until you educate yourself that you are what you eat. The problem isn't that we have an occasional hamburger, a slice of pizza, or a cup of ice cream. It's that we eat way too much of this stuff and not enough real food—fruits and vegetables. There must be a balance in our approach to eating. Moderation and management must take precedent over our cravings for more and more of the same old junk. Our health is at risk. Our children are at risk. Our economy is at risk. After all, someone pays for all of this. Eventually that someone is...*you*.

CHAPTER 5

Get Up, Get Moving, Get Better

...but bodily discipline is only of little profit, but godliness is profitable in all things, since it holds promise for the present life and also for the life to come. (1 Timothy 4:8)

My stepmother just turned the big "8-5" (in biblical terms that's "fourscore years" and five to grow on). "Mamaw," as she is affectionately known, is a marvelous lady and a blessing to a family left reeling in the wake of tragedy (the death of my mother to breast cancer in 1985). She put the sparkle back into our father's eye and has kept him going long after others would have given up. For her 85th birthday, Dad asked her what she would like to do. She smiled slightly and said, "I want to go to Wyoming and ride horses." So the two of them loaded up the Buick and headed west.

*Connie and Bobby...*For the record, *he* is Connie and *she* is Bobby. Named after the Philadelphia Athletics legendary baseball manager, Connie Mack (who won more baseball games than any manager in the history of Major League Baseball), my dad is a man's man. I suppose when you grow up with a name like "Connie" you have to be.

He called earlier this week to tell me they were staying on a ranch near Buffalo, Wyoming and had just come in from a two-hour trail ride. I asked how they were feeling, "Well, son, right now we're a bit bow-legged, but it's worth it considering all the wildlife we saw." You have to love it—eighty-five years young and still going strong. Bravo for them! It could be worse, I suppose. Former President Bush (#41) jumped out of airplanes to celebrate his octogenarian birthdays.

When our son, Dale, phoned his grandmother to wish her a happy birthday, she answered rather nonchalantly. "What are you doing, Mamaw?" he asked. "Oh, I'm sitting on a horse in the backcountry of Wyoming," she said with the same sort of voice inflection coming from someone who answered their phone while shopping at Wal-Mart. Dale was silent on the other end as he tried to assess the situation. "You answered your cell phone on the… back…of…a… horse?" "Sure, why not?" she replied. That's Mamaw.

They are amazing. In his book, *Echoes from the Nine Foot Road*, my father writes,

> "We meet many people who are much younger than we are and who suffer from poor health. Many younger people marvel at the schedule we keep. We don't stop to think about it much, we have been used to it for so long. Bobby can still outwork many women far younger than she. She can out walk me now. While I do stretch exercises every day, she does some which would put me in the hospital if I tried them. We both love to ride horses and do so at every opportunity. When we go on a trail ride, she tells the wrangler not to give her the slowest nag in the barn, but one with a little spirit. Neither of us takes much medication…"

Two things keep them going. First, a spiritual focus causes them to live each day without regret and as though it is their last. They read their Bibles daily and often together in the car as they travel. They are both people of prayer. They are well acquainted with the Book *and* its Author. Second, a regimen of personal self-discipline keeps them alive, alert, and sharp—both physically and mentally. They are avid early morning risers and often are up before the sun shines on the Kentucky bluegrass surrounding their Louisville home. They get out of bed, make it (a discipline instilled in me), and begin their exercise routine—she in one room and he in another. They proceed with a systematic twenty minute workout that may go longer if they hit the treadmill. On day-long car trips (which they take often) they'll stop at every other rest area to stretch and walk for fifteen to twenty minutes before proceeding on. At home, they break from the day's work and walk the neighborhood. They move. They eat right. They stay active. They attend functions. They never miss church assemblies. They go to bed early. They refuse to allow the effects of aging to turn them into rocking chair recluses. They are examples of the way it was intended to be.

And if you want to see my Dad bristle, ask him if he is "retired." You'll get an earful.

Someone asked when either my brother or I would advise them to "slow down." Here's the short version of the answer: Never. Why should we? They are having the time of their lives. May God increase their tribe. Better yet, I want to be *in* their tribe!

The Caleb-Man

His is one of the greatest stories in the Old Testament. Caleb first appears as one of the twelve leaders of Israel chosen by Moses and given the responsibility of exploring Canaan in anticipation of the God-led Hebrew invasion (Numbers 13-14). However, the report came back 10-2 in favor of the "giants" over Jehovah. And who were the two who rose above the mediocre majority? Joshua and Caleb. If you know the Old Testament; then you know the rest of the story. As punishment for their faithlessness, God postponed the Promised Land victory celebration for forty years until they learned their lesson and…until all the doubters died.

For forty years Caleb disappears from view. In Joshua 14, he resurfaces. He is now eighty-five years of age and just as feisty and faith-driven as ever. It is here that he gives one of the most passionate speeches you will ever read. Here it is…

> I was forty years old when Moses the servant of the LORD sent me from Kadesh-barnea to spy out the land, and I brought word back to him as it was in my heart. Nevertheless my brethren who went up with me made the heart of the people melt with fear; but I followed the LORD my God fully. So Moses swore on that day, saying, 'Surely the land on which your foot has trodden will be an inheritance to you and to your children forever, because you have

followed the LORD my God fully.' Now behold, the LORD has let me live, just as He spoke, these forty-five years, from the time that the LORD spoke this word to Moses, when Israel walked in the wilderness; and now behold, I am eighty-five years old today. I am still as strong today as I was in the day Moses sent me; as my strength was then, so my strength is now, for war and for going out and coming in. Now then, give me this hill country about which the LORD spoke on that day, for you heard on that day that Anakim [giants] were there, with great fortified cities; perhaps the LORD will be with me, and I will drive them out as the LORD has spoken. (Joshua 14:7-12)

He could have said, "Give me that rocking chair," or "Find me a soft, comfortable spot in the shade," or the familiar "I've done my part; it's time for the younger generation to take over..." But that's wouldn't have been Caleb. In fact; the last we see of him, he is walking up the hill, rolling up his sleeves, and readying himself to clear the giants from the land—*his* land. I venture to say there wasn't anyone big enough who wanted to tangle with the feisty eighty-five-year-old.

The Caleb-man is rare. And the reason is—most fail to forecast their lives into the eighth decade. However, the disciplines you engage in now will determine what kind of eighth decade you will have (or if you will have one at all). Hence, the "age old" question—"What do you want to be when you grow up—as in turning the big '8-5?'" I don't know about you, but riding horses in Wyoming sounds pretty good to me.

Sell the Barca-Lounger

Right about now I can hear someone quote 1 Timothy 4:8—"Bodily discipline [exercise] is only of little profit..." as a biblical excuse to sit down and rest in a rocker-recliner. That's not exactly an accurate exegesis of the verse. For one thing, the writer is comparing bodily discipline [exercise] to personal discipline [godly behavior]. For sure, the latter eclipses the former as priority one. Yet the latter doesn't mean the former isn't necessary. I knew an octogenarian weight lifter who loved to quote that verse and remind his students, "The Bible doesn't say exercise profits none. It's says it profits *little*. It's essential you get that 'little.'" Indeed.

While speaking in the Midwest, an older couple loaned me their car so I could visit a friend in a nearby town. A sticker on the bumper of their old Chrysler read, "Ask Me About My Barca-Lounger!" (my friend thought this was very funny). I think sometimes we have more "life rules" for older folks than we do for teenagers. We're always telling the older generation, "Watch out!" "Be careful!" "Slow down!" "Sit down and rest in this rocking chair…" *Really?* I love what Solomon said in Ecclesiastes 11:8—"Indeed, if a man should live many years, let him rejoice in them all" (11:8a). I don't know if Solomon had a bumper sticker on the royal chariot, but if he did, I think it would have read, "Ask Me How I Got Rid of My Barca-Lounger!"

God tells us in Psalm 90 that the scope of our life is "seventy years, or if due to strength, eighty years" (v.10). *If due to strength…* Listen, when God decides it's time for you to go home, He'll let you know. In the meantime, do not sit down. And throw away the word "retire." I don't care what the American mindset is about the magical age of sixty-five and this thing called "retirement." Even if the time comes for you to retire from the workforce, don't retire from "life force." Sadly, the following poem describes many…

> I get up each morning and dust off my wits.
> I pick up the paper and read the obits.
> If my name is missing, I know I'm not dead;
> So I eat a good breakfast and go back to bed.

Oh, brother.

I remember once asking my grandmother why she didn't hang out with those in her own age group. She answered without hesitation, "Most of those in my age group are in the cemetery and some that aren't ought to be!" That will give you some insight into her mindset. By the way, she always wanted to see Walt Disney World in Orlando, so I took her—*in her eighties.* We dined at the popular Contemporary Resort Hotel overlooking a beautiful Florida lake filled with ski boats racing from one end to the other. She said, "That looks like fun." Can you guess what we did next?

The story is told of a man who retired. Asked by a friend about his plans for first year, he replied: "I'm going to buy me a rocking chair." When asked about his plans for the second year, he replied: "Simple. I'm going to rock in it." Here's a P.S. for year number three: "You'll die in it!"

A study by one of the Ivy League schools followed two hundred people who retired at age sixty-five. Half of the group retired, settled into a rocking chair, and did nothing. The other half went immediately and either found other employment or poured themselves into a fascinating hobby that enabled them to maintain creativity, discipline, and usefulness. Guess what? The contrasts in the two groups were staggering. In fact, they found the probability of dying within ten years of the typical retirement age of sixty-five went up 500% for those who retired and did nothing. In other words, planning for the pasture can be dangerous to your health.

In 2003 I was hiking in Montana with several friends when we stopped for breakfast at a little Mom and Pop restaurant affixed to a gas station and not far from the trailhead. It was packed. In fact, it was packed with older men who weren't shy about introducing themselves or telling us about their hiking club. They met once a week for breakfast followed by a half-day hike in the woods. The club carried one stipulation: you had to be seventy-five to join. I learned about that rule from one of the hikers who subsequently smiled when I inquired about *his* age. "Ninety!" he said. "But I ain't 'bout to slow down."

None of these active seasoned seniors got to be that way overnight. They became that way because they made a decision to be that way. Years ago they found their turning point and determined to live within the boundaries of a healthy discipline—in other words; they disciplined their lives toward optimum health. And the time to begin that discipline is when you are young.

Some may conclude that such is radical. I guess it depends on one's definition of *radical*. If radical means stepping out from the ordinary and expected, then go for the radical. I love what Carter Hays says about the definition of "radical"—

> **Rad-i-cal:** An adjective (especially of change or action) relating to or affecting the fundamental nature of something.

> So, are you just…
> Going through the "motions" of life?
> Living in the "box of managed average" and BLAH?
> Reacting to change rather than orchestrating it?

Wondering what happens next?

"Wishing" things were better?

Well, jump in some ice water, stay there for 30 seconds
and become a "RADICAL" living person…

Enough is ENOUGH!
Become the Change.
Make things better.
Create "what" next.
Be the conductor.
Break down the wall of average, one wall at a time.
Create the "wake" on the lake.
Don't just go through the motions.

Spend one day, just one retooling your words by starting out with:
I AM radically _____!
You just don't have time to be complacent and take a moment off.
Never sell a minute of your day to "I don't know" or "Whatever?"
LIVE Radically.

That's great stuff. Living in the box of "managed average" is not what God expects from His people. Why would we want to follow the crowd when it comes to managing average? Look around. The crowd doesn't seem to be doing very well. Do you want better health than the "average?" Do you want to be ahead of the game when it comes to expecting the government to take care of you? Do you want to be alive, active, and available for your children's children? If so, you must make some radical (outside the ordinary) decisions—*now*.

Get Moving

The typical American way is to wait until you are unhealthy in order to get healthy. Why wait? Why not start *before* the "age thing" catches up with you so you can live life to the max for a long time? Take exercise, for example.

It's not what you think.

About now you expect me to quote the latest fitness guru's maxim on calorie burning that occurs through intense workouts. Some may need that in order to remain focused and to steer clear of old habits. There are plenty of articles, books, CD's, and DVD's that can give you the information needed for your particular situation. Above all, consult your physician for a plan of action. At the same time, some could benefit greatly from a qualified personal trainer who can provide both the information needed *and* hold you accountable. There is something to be said for the commitment of a financial investment. Like the old saying, "you get what you pay for." It's true.

Most of us, however, could profit greatly by engaging in moderate, consistent exercise that forces us off the couch and keeps both mind and muscle sharp. But that takes discipline and discipline means an investment called "time."

I have friends who love to run. I remember watching my brother run past me at mile marker 18 at Nashville's Country Music Marathon several years ago. I was there to cheer him on to the finish line (which was still over eight miles away). He came trotting past and didn't look anything like the spiffy fellow I had dropped off that morning near the Vanderbilt campus. The truth is, he looked like death. He saw me and said, "Go get the car! Go get the car!" That's a great line. By the way, he finished right at four hours. I asked him if those grueling 26.2 miles were worth it. "Absolutely!" he said. Then he added, "Few things are as exhilarating as training, competing, and crossing the finish line." Good for him.

I'd rather walk.

Because I travel a lot, I make a habit of walking four miles each day—and have done so for years. From the sidewalks of city streets to the wooded trails of national, state, and local parks, I hoof it. You don't need much equipment for that. In fact, you don't need much of a trail for that. Since I walk four miles per hour, I can walk in one direction for thirty minutes, turn around and come back. Easy. The hardest part is not the walking but the reprogramming of my mind that says this is something I must do daily.

My tennis shoes (I still call them *tennis* shoes—which is a misnomer because I don't play tennis) last about a year before I have a blow out. When I'm home, I walk the hour near the house. It's quiet. It's safe. It's country. There's nothing quite like walking on long cul-de-sacs in between white fencing in the midst of Tennessee horse country. Sure, I can walk on a treadmill (and I do sometimes when the weather is temperamental), but I prefer to be outside. For me, there is nothing as mind enhancing as an hour of brisk walking in God's world. I love it.

Do I miss a day now and then? Sure. Do I fret about missing a day now and then? No.

When it comes to exercise, the issue comes down to one thing: move. As in *move* off the couch and away from the desk. Move out of your Barca-Lounger, Lazy-Boy, or whatever else you tend to plop in. In fact, sell your Barca-Lounger on Craigslist! Then invest the money in good tennis (a-hem—*walking*) shoes.

Sherri Caldwell Nunley of Tampa, Florida has a B.A. in Wellness Leadership from the University of South Florida and has been a corporate exercise instructor for years—including employee fitness classes at Tampa General Hospital. Here's her take—

> Research shows that individuals choosing to lead an active lifestyle in their 40s live a healthier life in their older years. In my opinion, the key to staying fit is to find something you enjoy doing and decide to make it a habit. Finding the time of day that works best for you is also important. For me, exercising in the morning, before anyone else in the house gets up, gives me a chance to clear my head, think through the day's events and get my exercise behind me for the day. I have more energy and I feel better about myself. Because this is such a habit with me, I feel that as long as I am healthy and injury free, this lifestyle can help me through my later years.

I like simple. I like common sense. Sherri's approach is both.

Some buy treadmills, exercise bikes, and all sorts of equipment advertised on TV and designed to get you in shape in three easy payments (which aren't usually that easy). Exercise equipment ranks up there with travel trailers. It's the kind of thing that sounded like a good idea at the time. The truth is; they usually become very expensive towel hangers and/or clothes racks. That's what yard sales are for. Believe me; someone will buy your towel rack. Towel racks are in hot demand.

Dr. Logan Owens, PT, DPT, COMT, is the Memphis regional director for Results Physiotherapy. He knows about exercise and how it affects the body.

> The benefits from exercise are more than most realize. First, there is the obvious benefit of weight control and the decreased risk for high cholesterol, heart disease, type 2 diabetes, etc. Second, it helps with joint issues like osteoarthritis. Our joints are made up of bones lined in articular cartilage, surrounded by a capsule and filled with synovial fluid (think motor oil). Just as our body needs nutrition and energy, our joints need the same. And joints get nutrition from movement. Since bones grow based on the stresses we put on them, exercise strengthen them. Exercise also strengthens the muscles that support joints and the movement gives nutrients to the articular cartilage which typically doesn't have a strong blood supply.
>
> Improve blood flow and you improve oxygen distribution to the body. With improved oxygen to the body comes improved oxygen to the brain. There are so many benefits when it comes to exercise. When one of my patients concludes physical therapy, they are sent home with an exercise plan to maintain their improvement. Even in the case where a patient achieves 100% improvement, without maintaining the muscle strength and joint mobility going forward, they would not be able to keep the improvement they achieved.

In other words, keep moving. Your bones, brain, and body will thank you.

Like everything else, we tend to be very "gung-ho" about exercise at the beginning. However, if success is measured by the last thing you did (and it is) and the last thing you did was nothing—that doesn't exactly add up to much. Whatever you embark on as exercise routine, make it something you enjoy as much as you can. That doesn't mean you won't work and sweat like crazy. You will (if you don't, you're not exercising much of anything). But make a plan based on information from someone informed, and then execute the plan. Like anything else, if you want to make excuses that keep you from exercise, they are readily available. On the other hand, if you want to be eighty years old and riding horses in Wyoming or ninety years old and hiking in the Rockies, you've got to get in shape now. It won't happen by accident.

You Reap What You Sow

Carter Hays writes, "If we practice inconsistency, we will reap inconsistently." How true. He goes on to say, "To eat well occasionally, works well *occasionally*. To exercise every now and then works well *every now and then*. This is fine if you want a little bit of health a little bit of the time." Or how about this gem of wisdom from the same—

> Fictional fitness is like a book with hundreds of empty pages, producing nothing and simply a waste of time. Fictional fitness is empty promises that usually end in remorse and regret causing devastating health consequences. Get up. Get out. Get MOVING. And talk about it when you're done for the day!

How bad do you want to be healthy? Galatians 6:7 states the following law of creation: "You reap what you sow." And that's true in many areas. Yet the verse begins with a cautionary warning: "Do not be deceived..." Do you think he said that because maybe...it's easy to *be* deceived? And maybe...just maybe...the one we deceive most often is self?

Listen to Julie...

> You expect your heart to beat and keep up with all your activities. It is an organ made of muscle. And for it to be most effective, it must pump around 100,000 times per day. That's a lot of moving!

> Why do we expect less from all our other muscles? We sit, move slowly, and get annoyed when the word "exercise" is mentioned. I've been that way. I've never liked the word exercise; much less think it should be part of my daily living. Sigh. Just another thing to do!

> I've thought about what I encouraged through the years for my in-home patients to do who had been discharged from the hospital and were weak from illness. My first words were, "You need to move. Your muscles will get weak if you don't work them." And if they needed some help, I would have physical therapy ordered. I was right about that.

But I haven't always applied that rule to myself as a well person. And that has been a mistake. While my heart will "move" on its own without my telling it to, many other muscles, like in my arms and legs, depend on ME to put them into action. So why haven't I done a better job? Because I was doing what I "wanted" to do and not what I "needed" to do. That is the key to the total package... what you are thinking shows up in what you are doing.

My turning point was the realization that exercise is what my body needed so desperately and I had neglected it. My past was giving my body poor fuel and then letting it sit. That's an accident waiting to happen.

I wised up. I started "thinking" about what I do and quit giving in to those temptations that compel me to eat a donut, drink coffee and find a kind of comfort in that. My comfort now is knowing I can do this; I want to do this, and am taking care of myself; the kind of care that can only come from me!

When it comes to exercise most of us fall into two camps: (1) we love it, or (2) we hate it. Some suggest a third category: take it or leave it. But those folks almost always "leave it."

Dr. Ralph S. Paffenberger, physician at University of California at Berkeley stated, "We know that being physically fit is a way of protecting yourself against coronary heart disease, hypertension, and stroke, plus adult-onset diabetes, obesity, osteoporosis, probably colon cancer and maybe other cancers, and probably clinical depression. Exercise has an enormous impact on the quality of life" (as quoted in *Today Matters*, by John Maxwell, 96).

The problem with exercise is the same problem with making better eating choices. You don't receive immediate results. You exercise and weigh yourself. Nothing. The same routine is followed for days two and three. Still nothing. A week later, you've lost one or two pounds. Big deal. But it is a big deal because you are establishing a turning point for a healthier life. Eventually it will pay off in a very big way.

Like many things, the key is consistency. It's easy to exercise. However, it's easier not to exercise. The choice is in your head.

Yes, Today Matters

Mark Twain said this about procrastination: "Don't put off till tomorrow what may be done day after tomorrow just as well." A lot of us buy into that way of thinking. And while waiting until the last minute may allow you to squeak by with a "C" in American History, it won't allow for a passing grade when it comes to your health. Wait until the last minute and it may be your last minute.

I got up early this morning and found this on my Facebook page from Carter. "'I will' is the ultimate loss because you were never in the game in the first place. It is beyond my imagination to understand how someone can learn to do what they're not willing to do, yet complain that they couldn't do it." We've probably all been guilty.

In procrastination, we become our own worst enemy. And it's true in every area of life. We want our marriages to be better, yet put off taking the proactive steps to make it happen. We want our relationships with our children to become stronger, yet day after day goes by and nothing changes. We want to get a handle on our finances by reducing debt, yet those credit cards continue to be too much of a temptation. We want to know God better and get into His Word more regularly, yet another day of putting out the fires of the urgent have left us exhausted and spiritually empty. We want to lose weight, make better food choices, exercise and get in better shape physically, yet continue to find every reason (excuse?) why it isn't possible (at least not today). Tomorrow, we keep telling ourselves. Tomorrow will be different.

No it won't.

If you are waiting until tomorrow to do anything, you've already lost the battle. The battle is won on the day you set your face to do something about it. And that day is today.

My "today" came on my 55th birthday. I have been basking in the sunshine of "middle age" for years—even kidding an Alabama friend that I was still in the spring of life. "It must be a late spring this year," she replied.

Fifty-five... If fifty-five is middle age, then there must be some folks around here blowing out a hundred and ten birthday candles. Oddly enough, I can't find any.

I looked in the mirror on that day and said, "Enough." I needed to lose twenty pounds. It started that day. I needed to eliminate junk food. It started that day. I needed to stop drinking calories. It started that day. I needed to eat more fruits and vegetables. It started that day. I needed to lace up my shoes and hit the pavement. It started that day. That was months ago and each day is a reminder of that "mirror moment." I'm not looking back.

People create success by focusing on one day—*today*. You can study the lives of successful people and you will always find a common denominator: successful people make right decisions early and manage those decisions daily. Their daily agenda is not a long "to do" list. Rather, it is a lifestyle that is disciplined and prioritized. John Maxwell said, "You will never change your life until you change something you do daily. You see, success doesn't just suddenly occur one day in someone's life. For that matter, neither does a failure. Each is a process. Every day of your life is merely preparation for the next. What you become is the result of what you do today."

Maybe it's been a while since you wrapped your mind around the big picture. So here it is: you get one shot. It's called today—the *present* of the *present*. You will either focus on preparing yourself to be the best you can be—in relationships, finances, job performance, creativity, healthy choices, etc., or you will spend your final years focusing on repairing. Preparing or repairing? It's your choice. Sadly, most opt to spend their remaining days in repair mode—trying to fix what could have been avoided. It's a choice between the pain of self-discipline and the pain of regret.

It is said of Abraham that he "breathed his last and died in a ripe old age, an old man and satisfied with life" (Genesis 25:8). Abraham was committed to squeezing every drop out of life as long as he lived. So did Enoch (Genesis 5:24). So did Moses. So did Caleb. These people made the last years of their lives some of the best years of their lives. They stayed engaged. They stayed active. And they inspire me to do the same.

It's Easier to Maintain Your Health Than Regain Your Health

I love this Zig Ziglar quote. Zig asked: "If you had a million-dollar racehorse, would you allow it to smoke cigarettes, drink whiskey, and stay out all night? How about a thousand-dollar dog?" Obviously not. Anyone who has invested that much money into an animal would give it top-notch care—training, exercise, nutrition, etc. Okay (and you know where I'm going with this)—if you wouldn't allow your prized animal to do these things, then why would you allow yourself to do them?

Some become old long before their time (and die before their time) simply because they do not take care of themselves. Oddly enough, when we're young, we spend our health to get our wealth. Then in our latter years we reverse the order and spend our wealth to get our health. That's a whole lot of "spending" going on.

Here's a novel idea—why not spend time improving your health before it's too late? The key to your future health and well-being is to make the decision today to engage in common-sense disciplines that will be carried over to tomorrow and all the tomorrows after that. Like: eat healthier, drink more water, and exercise. No excuses.

As a southern boy at heart, I love fried chicken and banana pudding. After all, we're talking poultry and fruit, right? No one (including me) says that moderation isn't attainable. Thus I'll savor a piece of fried chicken and reward my taste buds with an occasional spoonful of banana pudding. But not overdo. What we often hear is: "But I get a craving for ____." Okay, let's put Blue Bell Rocky Road ice cream into the blank (yes, I know I need a longer blank for that to fit). You should know there are 320 calories in one cup of that delicious taste of Texas heaven. But who says you need to eat that much? The fact is: the recommended serving size is a half cup. I'm not good at math, but I think we just cut the calories down to 160. So enjoy an "occasional" scoop or two along with some berries and fruit. Eat less so you can enjoy more. Savor the treat. Your taste buds get their reward, your conscience can sleep, and you save money because you don't have to buy a bigger belt.

How about this—"My craving for life is greater than my craving for ___." The solution comes down to (1) moderation and (2) management. Eat smart, exercise, and watch the "feed limit."

A century ago the majority of sicknesses were related to infectious disease. Today they are related to poor eating choices and our sedentary lifestyles. And while you cannot go back and make a new start, you can start now and make a new end. But that depends on what you do today.

Hit the bricks. Go to the gym. Become accountable. Cut out the sugary drinks. Eat more good stuff and less "junk" stuff. However you do it—just do it!

Lace up those tennis shoes (*sneakers* if you're older than me—or *Keds* if you're a lot older than me) and get up, get moving, and get better.

CHAPTER 6

I Am Fearfully and Wonderfully Made

I will give thanks to You, for I am fearfully and wonderfully made;
Wonderful are Your works,
And my soul knows it very well. (Psalm 139:14)

There are some scenes that take your breath away and leave you at a loss for words. We were hiking in Glacier National Park near the Canadian border on a crisp, clear big-sky Montana day. There were ten of us—all guys from various occupations and professions. We had chatted off and on as we passed through heavy cedars while making the climb up the popular Avalanche Lake Trail. This is, after all, grizzly bear territory and hikers are "encouraged" to make their presence known. We were more than happy to oblige since grizzly bears outranked us on the food chain. As we approached the summit, the trail opened up into a wide vista that took in a greenish chilled iceberg lake surrounded by jagged peaks. Suddenly the chatter stopped. The silence was punctuated only by the howling wind that seemed to be trapped in the alpine bowl. As if on cue, each hiker distanced himself from the others. David, a surgeon, climbed onto a rock at water's edge and just sat and starred. A second Wilson, a retired captain with United Airlines (who documented the week's adventure through the lens of his camera), took no pictures. At that moment, and so mesmerized by what he saw, you knew he was capturing the scene through the lens of his eye and recording it forever in his mind. Another David (this one a

Kentucky lawyer friend), walked about seventy-five feet in one direction and I in another. No one spoke. No one had to. In fact, to do so would have seemed sacrilegious. Awed by the moment, we dared to take it in.

Have you seen Old Faithful? What about Niagara Falls? Or the Grand Canyon? What was your reaction? I hope you had one. And while people respond differently to emotional scenes—some with outside expressive emotions and others with an inward reflective quietness—you must respond. We must never allow ourselves to become calloused to the world around us. We must never lose our sense of amazement or awe at the touch of wonder experienced in God's magnificent world.

I love the story of the family with a nine-year-old boy who traveled across the country. His parents prepared him for the journey and even bought him a journal so he could write down his thoughts at what he saw along the way. Day after day they stopped at famous landmarks. Day after day he wrote nothing in his journal...until they got to Arizona and the Grand Canyon. He walked to the edge of that great chasm, peered across and then below, hesitated for a moment, and then raced back to the family minivan. He dug through his luggage until he found his journal. And then writing as fast as he could, he logged in his thoughts. The parents couldn't wait until bedtime when curiosity would lead them to open the book. When finally they did, this is the entry they found: "Today is the best day of my life. Today I spitted a mile!" Kids, you gotta love 'em.

By nature children are governed by the touch of wonder. Kids, after all, have to touch and experience everything. A simple rock becomes a touch of wonder to be guarded and treasured. After all, there will never be another rock like this one. A leaf, a shell, a bug—touch of wonders, all. Give a kid the choice between a fistful of dandelions for his mother and a dozen roses, he chooses the bright yellow flowers every time. And what mom doesn't treasure them more than all the roses in the world.

The problem is this: we grow up. We leave the world of childhood innocence where everything is awe-inspiring and amazing and enter the cold, practical, and matter-of-fact world of sterile adulthood. We walk into an environment of scientific explanations, assembly lines, interchangeable parts, computer screens, deadlines, traffic jams, and...suddenly it's gone.

Poof! Exit wonder and enter the monotonous boredom of sameness. Occasionally we are reminded to "stop and smell the roses," but who really has the time? We lose the touch of wonder and lose our sense of awe.

David never did. In the 139th Psalm, a song tucked away in the ancient hymnal of Israel, the former shepherd-turned-giant-slayer-turned-king records what happens when a human being stops long enough to think about God, himself, and the amazing world of which he is a part. The song has four stanzas—each touching on the wonders of God.

I know. I know. You're asking, *what does this have to do with health, happiness, and physical wholeness?* Everything! You do not exist in a vacuum. You exist for a reason. And until you gain a sense of the human experience from every vantage point—physical, mental, emotional, and spiritual—you will never have the resolve to live to your peak level of human potential. So, stay with me…

The Wonder of God's Knowledge

In verses 1-6, David describes the all-knowing God. Please note that the author isn't describing God's knowledge in an abstract and philosophical way but in a close and personal way. "O Lord, You have searched **me** and known **me**" (v.1). David is stopped in his tracks at the thought that the Creator of the universe, the One who controls the heavens and rules the world—knows *me*. He knows…*me?* Yes. In fact, He not only *knows* you, He cares deeply about you. That's why Peter said to cast "all your anxiety on Him, because He cares for you" (1 Peter 5:7). Jesus even said, "the hairs of your head are numbered" (Matthew 10:30). The point? God knows everything about you. In fact, He knows you better than you know you.

Why is this important to know? Because…the next time you have a down day, or someone tries to steal your self-worth, or the next time someone can't remember your name—it doesn't matter. Look at the beautiful magnificent world of which you are a part and wrap your arms around this living thought: the God who did all of this—*knows and cares about me!*

If that isn't incentive enough to cause you to present back to the Creator the best you that you can be, I'm at a loss as to any better motivation behind physical stewardship (the taking care of your body).

What specifically does God know about me?

- **He knows what I do.** "You know when I sit down and when I rise up," v.2a. The words "sit down" are passive while the words "rise up" are active. It is a Hebrew phrase denoting the day-to-day activities of life (Deuteronomy 6:7). From rest to work, God knows and cares about every part of your day.

- **He knows what I think.** "You understand my thought from afar," (v.2b). We may disguise our self-defeating thoughts from friends and family, but God knows. He is well acquainted with your self-talk. He knows what you say and He knows why you are saying it.

- **He knows where I go.** "You scrutinize my path and my lying down, and are intimately acquainted with all my ways," (v.3). God knows your path—and He knows when that path is on the straight and narrow and when it's leading you back to the old playground that got you into trouble. Art Adams, an addiction counselor for the state of Indiana, tells his audiences that to break free from any addiction requires three changes. "You have to change your playground, your playmates, and your playthings." In other words, the places, people, and things that got you to this point in life must be changed. It's a hard and fast rule with no excuses. You cannot return to what got you into trouble. And God knows. God knows when you're sticking with the new you and/or when you are tempted to cheat. He is "intimately acquainted" with you.

- **He knows what I say.** "Even before there is a word on my tongue, behold, O Lord, you know it all," (v.4). Even the words you tell yourself are no secret to Him.

- **He knows what I need.** "You have enclosed me behind and before, and laid your hand upon me," (v.5). God protects you, provides for you, and pushes you along. The point? God is there for you every step of the way.

And what is David's reaction to this incredible realization about God? "Such knowledge is too wonderful for me; it is too high, I cannot attain it," (v.6). Try as you might, the finite you cannot wrap your mind around the infinite Him. At the end of the day, like David, we merely confess it (even though we don't understand it). Paul summed it up in Romans 11:33—"Oh, the depths and the riches both of the wisdom and knowledge of God! How unsearchable are His judgments and unfathomable are His ways!" Try as we might to grasp and articulate God's greatness; it is an impossible task. As a result, we merely stand in awe.

The Wonder of God's Presence

The atheist professor had written this declaration on the board:

GOD IS NOWHERE.

Upon arrival the next day, a creative student had made the following subtle change:

GOD IS NOW/HERE.

Likewise, in the second stanza (vv.7-12), David turns his thoughts to the omnipresence of God and confesses that the Creator is not limited by distance or by time. Verse 7—"Where can I go from Your Spirit? Or where can I flee from Your presence?" It's not that David is wanting to escape from God, but merely is confessing the futility of the very thought.

I was teaching a class of small children several years ago when I asked the question: "Is there any place you can go where God isn't?" The kids all thought for a moment (you could see the miniature wheels turning) and then one little boy's hand shot in the air. Excitedly he proclaimed, "New Jersey!" I asked him why he thought God wasn't in New Jersey. He responded by saying that his father had gone to New Jersey and had been heard mumbling something about "this God-forsaken place." Hmm. Kids indeed say the craziest things. That's why teachers of children learn to smile and move on. And just for the record, I've been to New Jersey and… God is there, too.

What is the message of the book of Jonah if it is not punctuated by the theme that you can't run away from God? And in one of the most bizarre scenes in the opening pages of Scripture, God walks among the foliage of the Garden while Adam and Eve were hiding behind a tree. *Really?* God asked Jeremiah (23:24), "Can a man hide himself in hiding places so I do not see him?" Uh, no.

David confesses two truths in verse 8—"If I ascend to heaven, You are there; if I make my bed in Sheol [the realm of the dead], behold, You are there." From the heights of the heavens to the depths of the earth, God is there. He further states, "If I take the wings of the dawn, if I dwell in the remotest parts of the sea, even there Your hand will lead me, and Your right hand will lay hold of me" (vv.9-10). Think: if somehow you could travel at the speed of light, you could not outrun God. Or if you could descend to the deepest and darkest level of the ocean, you could not escape Him. Heights or depths, land or sea, it doesn't matter. God is there.

"If I say, 'Surely the darkness will overwhelm me, and the light around me will be night,' even the darkness is not dark to You, and the night is as bright as the day. Darkness and light are alike to You," (vv.11-12).

I recall with fondness my grandparent's country home in Virginia that backed up to the woods and was surrounded by the biggest oak trees I have ever seen. As the sun set and dusk descended, we played hide-and-go-seek until we could see no more. The cover of darkness only made it more adventuresome. I could hide and no one could see me. It's funny how darkness makes us think we are invincible. That why some continue to play in their own little hide-and-seek world of make-believe by thinking they can escape the eye of God. You can't. "And there is no creature hidden from His sight, but all things are open and laid bare in the eyes of Him with whom we have to do" (Hebrews 4:13).

While the nearness of God can be terribly frightening to one who lives outside of His directives, it is a comfort to those who seek His favor and friendship. "Do not fear, for I am with you. Do not anxiously look about you, for I am your God. I will strengthen you, surely I will help you, surely I will uphold you with My righteous right hand" (Isaiah 41:10). What a comfort that is to me—and I hope to you, too.

The Wonder of God's Power

Stanza three focuses on God's unlimited power. And while several scriptures point to His power in the creation of the universe (Psalm 19:1—"the heavens are telling of the glory of God"); David zooms in on the wonder of birth and the awe of human life. Conception, the development of a child in the womb, and the marvel of birth are certainly wonders that no study of genetics, anatomy, or obstetrics can possibly erase.

I must tell you that I have a very hard time with those who view an unborn child as a mere extension of tissue or something akin to an appendix. David reminds us that God is the author of life. And he makes it clear that the Creator is personally involved with the development of each child.

"For You formed my inward parts; You wove me in my mother's womb," (v.13). Who did the forming? Who did the weaving? God did. "Before I formed you in the womb I knew you," said God to the prophet Jeremiah (1:5). Isaiah confessed the same and gave God the glory for his development and birth (Isaiah 49:5). In Matthew 1:18, Mary was said to be "with child." It is a child in the womb of the mother and a child who is carefully made unique and unlike any other.

You've heard it said that there are no two snowflakes alike. That's a big deal and amazing phenomena. Okay, here's a much bigger deal: out of all the billions of people who have walked on this planet, there are no two people alike! The DNA of each person is absolutely unique. Ask the parents of identical twins if they are really identical. They aren't. Their physical features may be the same, but there are marked differences. Think about your children. I doubt this is much of a stretch, but I will hazard the guess that they are each very different. Undoubtedly that's ditto for you and your siblings, too.

I have one brother and we aren't anything alike. He's short and I'm tall. He's bald and I'm still holding on (of course, he's quick to remind me that they don't put marble tops on cheap furniture!). He's smart (this is where the analogy takes a very bad turn) and I'm…well, never mind. Seriously, he took courses I couldn't even pronounce—and aced them. My brother had the most boring report cards ever: "A," "A," "A,"—ad nauseum. Okay, at least mine had variety. Pick a letter of the alphabet and it was probably there.

The point? We are all different. In fact, we are all *very* different. And who is responsible for the unique differences? God. All of which says we need to stop trying to be everyone else and start trying to be the best person God created us to be. We must learn to value our uniqueness and develop our strengths rather than crying over our limitations. Determine to be the *best* you that you were created to be.

"I will give thanks to You, for I am fearfully and wonderfully made" (v.14a). There is no place where the power of God is seen with greater clarity than in the creation and development of human life. Those who fain disbelief in God have yet to come to terms with the complexities of the human body. For example, there is no computer that can do what the human mind can do—and for the length that it can function. Technology, on the other hand, has a window of viability that is very small. It's been said that as soon as you get it home from the store, it's obsolete. That's pretty close to accurate. At the same time, no camera can record all that the eye can see and store it to be replayed again and again. Is all of this by mere chance?

My friend has a meticulously restored 1967 Chevrolet Camaro. It's the kind of dream car that leaves your mouth open and drooling. Just don't drool on the car! What do you think would happen if he tried to convince me that his car came together as the result of a huge explosion in his garage and that all the pieces just fell into perfect position? Yeah, right. Nobody in their right mind would buy that. And yet the same logic (?) is applied to the question of human origin by men of great "learning" and we shake our heads and say, "Wow, that's really profound!" It's not profound at all. In fact, it's quite the opposite.

David was quick to give God the glory and the credit. "Wonderful are Your works, and my soul knows it very well," (v.14b).

Your body—your physical self—is a testimony to the power and creativity of God. He has presented you with the gift of life and asks that you treasure the gift. You have one incredible body that is capable of amazing things, but only if you value it and take care of it. It is designed to last seventy to eighty years and beyond, but not if you abuse it. Solomon said, "put away pain from your body" (Ecclesiastes 11:10). *Don't do anything that will destroy, diminish, or damage your physical self.* And for two reasons: (1) it is God's gift to you, and (2) you only have one. Take care of it so that you can offer your best back to Him and the people He places in your life. Paul said your body is a "temple of the Holy Spirit who is in you, whom you have from God, and that you are not your own..." (1 Corinthians 6:19). The principle of stewardship is alive and well when it comes to the physical conditioning of your body. That's why he goes on to say, "Glorify

God in your body" (v.20). Use what He has given you in the best and healthiest way you can. Settle for nothing less.

David isn't done. He adds, "My frame was not hidden from You, when I was made in secret, and skillfully wrought in the depths of the earth," (v.15). It's a poetic description of the developing child in the womb. Your "frame" references your skeletal structure; your bones. "Skillfully wrought" is a reminder that God put you together with His touches of TLC. You are no accident. You are the product of a loving God who made you one of a kind.

"Your eyes have seen my unformed substance; and in Your book were all written the days that were ordained for me, when as yet there was not one of them," (v.16). Think of the excitement the first time you laid eyes on your newborn. In fact, you couldn't take your eyes off him/her. You counted toes and fingers. You spotted unique markings that looked familiar—"He has his daddy's eyes…" "She has her momma's nose…" Remember? There is nothing like those first moments of birth as parents are struck with the awe and wonder of human life. God, however, saw you from the moment of conception. He watched you take shape, grow, and form. He stitched your personality and wove your neurological threads completely different that anyone else's. He made you uniquely you.

Consider ten amazing facts about your physical body (gathered from various sources):

- If the blood vessels in your body were placed end to end, they would circle the earth with a length of 25,000 miles. Are you kidding me? No.

- Your lungs alone contain 300,000 million blood vessels. If laid end to end, they would stretch 1,500 miles.

- Human bone is four times as strong as concrete. One cubic inch of your bone can support 8.6 tons.

- Each kidney contains one million individual filters. They filter approximately 2.2 pints of blood per minute and expel 2.5 pints of urine per day.

- The muscles in your eyes move approximately 100,000 times per day.

If you were to give your leg muscles the same amount of exercise, you would need to walk fifty miles each day.

• You shed over forty pounds of skin in your lifetime. Hmm. I'm not sure I want to think much about this one. Of course, it could be worse seeing that snakes shed their skin all at once. Imagine walking around and finding "people skin" everywhere. (Okay, let's not imagine that).

• You will produce enough saliva in your life to fill two swimming pools.

• Your nose can detect more than 50,000 different scents.

• The air from your sneeze travels over 100 miles per hour.

• And…for every pound of fat you gain, your body compensates by laying down seven new miles of blood vessels. All of which means your heart must work even harder to pump blood through all these new avenues (which strains your entire grid system). The good news: for every pound of fat you lose, your body will reabsorb the now unnecessary vessels. And that means: less infrastructure = better health!

Talk about a WOW FACTOR! Our bodies reflect an amazing design and durable function over an incredible long period of time. No wonder David exclaimed, "I am fearfully and wonderfully made." Indeed.

And what is David's reaction as he ponders the mysterious event called human life? Praise! "How precious also are Your thoughts to me, O God! How vast is the sum of them! If I should count them, they would outnumber the sand. When I am awake, I am still with You," (vv.17-18). Note: it's not what David thought about God that stirred his emotions, but the fact that God thought that much of Him! Standing beneath a canopy of stars, the same David asked in Psalm 8, "What is man that You take thought of Him?" It's a good question. The answer is made plain in Scripture. God says, in essence, *Look around… Do you see all of this? I did it all for…you!* Do you "get it?" Do you understand how unique you are and… how special you are to Him?

The Wonder of God's Judgment

The fourth stanza seems out of place (vv.19-22). This final section must be read with an understanding of who David was—a theocratic king appointed by God, ruling for God, and responsible to God. These are not the words of personal malice and individual vindictiveness, but the words of a king jealous for His God. He is asking God to judge his enemies—because they were God's enemies. He is concerned about God's holy name. He is concerned about God's holy people. But in the end he returns to himself (vv.23-24):

> Search me, O God, and know my heart;
> Try me and know my anxious thoughts;
> And see if there be any hurtful way in me,
> And lead me in the everlasting way.

God's king was grieved at the evil deeds of the wicked. Yet, at the same time, David wanted to make sure that his own life did not grieve his Maker. "Search *me*..." "Try *me*..." "Lead *me*..." It's easy to point the finger of accusation at others (and there are times when we must hold others accountable). But at the end of the day and at the end of life, each is responsible for his own life. And on that day, God, the ultimate Judge of human life, will not ask us what we think about Mary or John, Sue or Bob... His concern will be about one human being: *you*. Did you take the time to recognize Him and the power of His creation? Did you treasure the gift of His precious Son? Did you respond in loving obedience to Him? And did you value the gift of the one life He gave you? What kind of steward were you with what He allowed you to have?

Final Thoughts

Years ago some pranksters snuck into a department store. Rather than stealing anything, they engaged in mischief-making. And here's what they did. They went throughout the store and rearranged all the price tags (this was obviously in the days before computers and bar codes). They took tags from cheaper merchandise and placed them on expensive items and vice-versa. The odd thing is, the store opened the next morning and functioned normally for two hours before anyone caught on. Some got great deals while others got ripped off.

Don't look now, but someone may have exchanged your price tag! You were created as a one-of-a-kind, priceless, human being. You were designed by the One who placed the stars in the heavens and who made the earth perfectly suited to support life. Everything He made, He made for you. That's why you must never doubt your worth in His eyes. You are, in fact, the apple of His eye.

Remember that the next time someone tries to hang you with a bargain-basement price tag or the next time you are tempted to give in to self-defeating thoughts. One of the common refrains of those who succumb to addictive behavior is that they feel completely worthless. They allow themselves to be measured by others instead of being measured by the God who made them and put them here for a reason.

You are one incredible person.

You are here on this planet for a purpose.

You are the reason for it all.

You are fearfully and wonderfully made.

And don't *you* ever forget it.

CHAPTER 7

Modern Day Marlboro Men (and Women)

Or do you not know that your body is a temple of the Holy Spirit
who is in you, whom you have from God, and that you are not
your own? For you have been bought with a price; therefore
glorify God in your body. (1 Corinthians 6:19-20)

I am a baby boomer child of the 50s and 60s. It was a different era
and one that, in many ways, seems foreign to the world of today. I've
often wondered what would happen if you stuck a kid in a time machine
and sent him back for a day. That would be interesting. "Hey, where's
the remote?" "Why is tin foil hanging on the TV antenna?" (Then again,
"What's an antenna?") "What's this round-rotary looking thing on the
phone?" "What do you mean you don't have a computer?" And..."How
come everybody's smoking?"

Funny questions—until you ask the last one.

Post-World War II America was an idyllic time of simplicity and prosperity.
We stopped making tanks and war planes and started making Fords and
Frigidaires. And we made a lot of them. People were happy with all the
new modern inventions and conveniences—instant coffee, TV dinners,
supermarkets, air-conditioning, and automatic transmissions.

We were also happily indestructible. We didn't wear seat belts, have air

Turning Point

bags, or have to replace the batteries in our smoke detectors. Come to think of it, we didn't have smoke detectors. Neither did we have child-safety caps on medications. Kids didn't wear helmets when they rode a bicycle or pads for their knees when they were skating (they would have been laughed off the playground). In fact, we did both—*in the street.* And we had no cell phones to report on our whereabouts. We did know the boundaries and we knew to be home at 5:00 for supper (or else there would be no supper). Somehow we survived.

And we certainly didn't worry about the foods we ate because we knew the food companies only made food that was good for us. We were given sugar for energy, red meat to make us strong, and ice cream for healthy bones. Oh, yes, we ate a lox of wax candy—especially those wax miniature pop bottles where you would drink a small amount of colored liquid that tasted like transmission fluid and then you would chew the wax for the rest of the day. What blissful fun!

In many ways it was the age of endearing innocence. Or was it stupidity?

Take nuclear bombs, for example. Every few weeks at Voris Elementary School in Akron, Ohio (where we lived for a few years in the 60s), we would have a civil defense drill. There would be a siren indicative of a Russian invasion of some sort, and all the kids in Mrs. Johnson's fifth grade class would leave their seats and get under their desks. We were instructed to fold our hands over our head and remain in the nuclear attack brace position until the all-clear was sounded. Decades later I am struck by two things (and neither one a missile). First, that a little wooden school desk would shield anyone from a nuclear attack seems a bit of a stretch. Second, that the Russians would bomb Akron seems even more so.

Welcome to the completely oblivious, happy-go-lucky 50s and 60s.

And of course, we smoked. Most everybody did. Cigarettes, we were told, actually made you healthier. Fact is, the advertisers promised us they would soothe nerves and sharpen minds. An ad for L & M cigarettes in *The Journal of the American Medical Association* (where cigarette ads were welcomed into the 50s and 60s) read, "Just what the doctor ordered!" A popular ad for the Camel brand showed a doctor in his lab coat with a stethoscope around his neck while holding a cigarette. The caption read: "More Doctors Smoke Camels Than Any Other Cigarette!" The copy beneath the ad said, "This is no casual claim. It's an actual fact. Based on the statements of doctors themselves to three nationally known independent research organizations." Not to be outdone, Lucky Strikes came out with their own doctor ad showing a smiling physician and copy that read: "20,679 Physicians Say LUCKIES Are Less Irritating." It makes you wonder how many of the 20,679 died of lung cancer.

Thus, if it was good enough for the doctors, it was good enough for the rest of us.

My grandfather on my mother's side smoked. No one thought a thing about it. The men at church would go out the back or side door (sometimes the front door) and smoke between Sunday School and worship. No one thought a thing about it. We rode in buses full of smoke, flew in airplanes full of smoke, ate in restaurants full of smoke, and watched movies in smoked-filled theaters. Were we naïve? Yes. Did we care? No.

Fast forward fifty years and the public perception of smoking has changed radically. It hasn't happened quickly, but generationally. As more and more medical studies were concluded, it became obvious that, contrary to what the tobacco companies had been telling us, cigarettes were not only bad for our health, they were, in fact, killing us. It took a while, but we finally caught on. We had been duped.

The Marlboro Man

When tobacco giant Phillip Morris introduced the Marlboro Man, they turned the Marlboro brand into the top-selling cigarette in the world (where it remains today). The Marlboro Man exemplified manhood— freedom, outdoor ruggedness, along with the cowboy mystique of the great American West. Three men appeared in the Marlboro ads over the years and all three died of...lung cancer. But America didn't seem to notice (or didn't want to notice). Today the Marlboro brand is alive and well and, like its competitors, is marketed around the world. While smoking has declined in the U.S. (approximately 19% of Americans currently smoke), it has increased in other countries. It is estimated that 50% of the men in

China smoke. In the Middle East, Latin America, Africa, and some parts of Europe, smoking is in vogue and on the increase.

The first Surgeon General's warning linking cigarettes to health issues was issued in 1964. A rather bland message appeared on cigarettes that read, "Caution: Cigarette Smoking May Be Harmful to Your Health." It was quite ineffective and carried about as much weight as a sign at the entrance to a swimming pool that said "Swim At Your Own Risk." By 1972, a new label appeared, although tucked neatly on the side of the pack, which was also vague and hard to read. It said, "Warning: The Surgeon General Has Determined That Cigarette Smoking Is Dangerous To Your Health." Today the warning labels are much more informative and rotate among the following messages:

SURGEON GENERAL WARNING:
Cigarette Smoke Contains Carbon Monoxide

SURGEON GENERAL WARNING:
Smoking Causes Lung Cancer, Heart Disease, Emphysema, and May Complicate Pregnancy

SURGEON GENERAL WARNING:
Smoking By Pregnant Women May Result In Fetal Injury, Premature Birth, and Low Birth Weight

SURGEON GENERAL WARNING:
Quitting Smoking Now Greatly Reduces Serious Risks To Your Health

By 1971, it became illegal for tobacco companies to advertise cigarettes on radio or television. In the 1980s, even Hollywood contributed efforts to anti-smoking campaigns. By the 1990s, the tobacco companies settled a huge lawsuit brought by the attorney generals of 46 states and the District of Columbia (Florida, Minnesota, Texas, and Mississippi had already reached an agreement with the tobacco industry) which forced them to pay states annually to compensate for medical costs related to treating citizens with tobacco-related illnesses. It was the biggest legal settlement in U.S. history. Eventually smoking was banned on all commercial airline flights (1998). When it became apparent that second-hand smoke was just as hazardous, many states and local jurisdictions passed smoking bans in all enclosed locations and in many outdoor venues, including sport stadiums.

Today we lead healthier lives due to education and information about the dangers of cigarette smoking. It didn't happen overnight, but gradually we caught up to the learning curve. And while smoking remains an issue in some places, those desirous of better health have responded with overwhelming approval.

Yet in spite of settling huge lawsuits, companies such as Phillip Morris and R.J. Reynolds continue to be profitable due to the increase in smoking worldwide. Phillip Morris is so profitable, in fact, that it continues to diversify. Phillip Morris first diversified in the 1960s when it purchased the Miller Brewing Company. In more recent times it has entered the processed food industry with the acquisition of General Foods and Kraft. According to Moss, "ten cents of every dollar an American spends on groceries now belongs to Phillip Morris." In fact, food has not only overtaken cigarettes as their largest division, Phillip Morris has become the largest food company in the country. Think about that the next time you buy Cool Whip, Oscar Mayer, Lunchables, Shake 'n' Bake, Velveeta, Jell-O, Maxwell House, Raisin Bran, Grape Nuts, Cocoa Pebbles and dozens of other popular sellers.

This doesn't mean that a consumer should support only those companies with whom they are in complete agreement on every issue (good luck with that!) any more than they should not pay taxes to a corrupt government that misspends money. Such would be impossible. Jesus understood the principle that all of us live in the world (Matthew 22:21; John 17:15)—which isn't a problem unless we allow the world to start living in us.

It does, however, argue one thing: big tobacco is still big tobacco and now…processed foods.

Back to the Future

In many ways we have reverted back to the "hear no evil, see no evil" innocence of the 50s and 60s. Only this time the issue isn't nuclear bombs or cigarettes—it's junk food. So, our twenty-first century kids sit safely buckled in their approved child safety seats surrounded by air bags while we wait in the drive-thru to obtain a sack full of who knows what. Yes, we've come so far from where we've been that we're back to where we started. Good ol' American inconsistency.

Take food warning labels—uh, I mean, "nutrition labels." While the nutrition labels on processed foods in the grocery store are there for us to read, we either don't read them or don't want to read them. Once more, we have gone back to the future and entered the ignorance-is-bliss zone.

In 1990, the Nutrition Labeling and Education Act was passed requiring all packaged foods to carry nutrition labels. As a consumer, you can read them or ignore them (in much the same way as people read or ignored cigarette warning labels). You *can* educate yourself about food labels and what they mean. You *can* know what you are putting into your one-and-only body and the bodies of your children. At the same time, the principle of moderation comes into play. We can become so over-the-top consumed with label reading that we lose all sense of balance (not to speak of time in the grocery store aisle). Like most things, the answer is not in extremes but in educating ourselves to make better choices. And while we don't have to smoke, we do have to eat. But in so doing, we need to feed ourselves more *real* food and less *junk* food. Or in the words of popular author David Zinczenko, "Eat This, Not That!"

A quick glance at a nutrition facts label will reveal the following...

SERVINGS. This is usually at the top of the label and one of the first things you see. Yet, this is where food companies love to trick us. Welcome to the world of...*portion distortion.* Americans tend to overeat by thinking that everything in the package counts as one serving. Not so fast, Mr. and Mrs. Consumer. Read the *servings per container.* Many times it will say 2 or 2.5 servings. This is where that middle school math comes in handy—as in basic multiplication. Two servings mean that I either (1) eat only half of the food, or (2) multiply all those numbers on the label by two.

Note to self: By throwing "Low-Cal!" or something similar and splashy on the packaging, food companies hope you will be so impressed that you won't notice that the package in your hand contains multiple servings. You can, however, outsmart the food companies, but only if you read the label.

CALORIES. The number given doesn't translate into whatever you want to eat. It's the number of calories *per serving.* Once again, break out the calculator.

SUGAR. This bad-boy number is accompanied by the letter "g." It stands for "grams." Think of it this way: four grams of sugar equal one sugar cube. For example, one serving of General Mills Trix cereal contains twelve grams of sugar—the equivalent of three sugar cubes. On the other hand, a Cinnabon Cinnamon Roll contains...*drum roll*...55 grams of sugar. Eat one and it's the same as crunching on 14 sugar cubes. No wonder they're so good!

Note to self: If you read the small print "ingredients" and come across stuff like "high fructose corn syrup"—that's sugar, too. As Bob Harper says, "If it [high fructose corn syrup] appears in the first five ingredients, keep walkin.'"

SODIUM. We need salt, just not as much as we normally eat. If you are in good health, keep it in the 2,000-2,400mg per day range. If you read the labels, it will blow your mind how quickly the sodium numbers add up. However, if you do not read the labels, the numbers (ahem...*pounds*) will add up even quicker.

TOTAL FAT. Fat is not a bad thing (saturated fat *is* a bad thing) since, like salt, we need some in our diet. Harper's book, *Skinny Rules*, says, "The label will tell you the percentage of fat calories per serving. *If it is over 20%, walk away.*"

FIBER. The more the merrier. This is one ingredient we don't get enough of. By the way, fruits and vegetables are loaded with fiber. The trick? Eat more fruits and vegetables.

Note to self: Fruits and vegetables are *real* food. (Duh!)

There is a lot of other information on there, and you can research the information and what it means via an internet search. Remember this: the fine print "ingredients" will list everything contained in the product. You will want to read that too, although you may need some high-powered magnifying glasses to do so. Like legalese in a contract, it's in extra small print for a reason. Some companies hope you won't notice. It's like the lady who read the ingredient list to find that the food product she was purchasing contained "Carnauba wax." Carnauba wax is what gives floors and shoes their shine. She concluded that while Carnauba wax might be okay for floors and shoes, it wasn't an okay ingredient to feed her kids. Smart mom. (I was taking my car through one of those automatic car washes last week and noticed a big flashing sign that said, "Now Applying Carnauba Wax!" Do you really want to eat that?)

Here are three common-sense rules of thumb:

Thumb rule #1: If you can't pronounce it, you probably shouldn't eat it. Many of those science-sounding words are chemicals that preserve the shelf life of the food. Some processed foods contain enough preservatives to give them a shelf life for a year. That's good for *shelf* life, but not always good for *your* life.

Thumb Rule #2: Watch out for the word "imitation." It means what it says. For example, "imitation cheddar cheese" means it's not cheddar cheese. Each time you read "imitation," substitute the word "fake" (as in "fake" food). Somehow "fake food" doesn't sound nearly as good as the euphemistic "imitation." Sometimes you may even read the words, "Real Imitation…" Think about that one.

Thumb Rule #3: The more items in the ingredient paragraph, the more processed it is, and the more processed it is, the less excited you should be about it.

Will Junk Food be the Next Tobacco?

If the junk food lifestyle of Americans is bad, that of the Brits may be even worse. The National Health Service (NHS) in Britain has reported that disease caused by unhealthy eating habits has overtaken those caused by cigarettes or alcohol. A study by Oxford University says obesity and poor diet now place "the largest economic burden" upon the health-care system. In a story by Laura Donnelly, health correspondent with Telegraph Media, she reports a spokesperson from the National Obesity Forum as saying, "The costs [associated with obesity] are staggering—this is bringing the NHS to its knees."

When fried, fatty, sugary, and salty foods become the staple of our diet, it should come as no surprise when health costs soar. And while all things in this comparison (junk food versus cigarettes) are **not** equal, some of them are and are worth a measured consideration.

- **Both make you sick.** It's no longer a secret that cigarettes contribute to cancer in various forms as well as to heart disease. Obesity also leads to heart disease, diabetes, kidney failure and other health-related issues. And what is the leading cause of obesity? Junky, processed foods.

- **Both are addictive.** By now everyone understands that nicotine in cigarettes is addictive. Studies show that processed foods high in sugar, fat, and salt trigger similar addiction-like responses. That's why those with a diet of junk food, often "crave" more of the same. Like other euphemisms, "crave" sounds less harsh and judgmental than an evil word like "addiction."

- **Both are regulated.** Cigarettes are obviously regulated more than food. But even that did not happen quickly or without smokers howling about (1) overreaction, (2) media hysteria, and (3) too much government control (sound familiar?). Even non-smokers thought such was intrusive until...they learned that "second hand smoke" caused them to get sick, too. Suddenly, we were "all in." At one point, half of all adults in the U.S. smoked. That number has been reduced to a nationwide average of 19% (the tobacco–producing state of Kentucky leads the nation as the "smokiest" state with 28%, followed by West Virginia with 27%, and Oklahoma with 25%. On the other hand, Mormon-populated Utah has the least smokers at 11%). A similar thing is happening when it comes to junk food. Until now, Joe Public has taken the stance that overeating junk hurts only the one who so indulges. Yet when health care costs are sent spiraling out of control and the medical bills are passed along to everyone (including raising *Joe's* health insurance premiums), suddenly it's a whole new ballgame. We're wising up and figuring out that unhealthy food choices eventually affect everyone—in the pocketbook.

John Banzhaf is one of the attorneys who sued big tobacco in the 60s. He is a law professor at George Washington University and founder of

Action on Smoking and Health. "Those legal actions against smoking had a lot to do with changing the mind of the public. In the fifties, sixties, seventies, eighties, even early nineties, most people blamed smoking solely on the smoker. It was his fault, it was his bad choice, it was his lack of responsibility" (quoted in *Obsessed* by Mika Brzezinski). Truthfully, it was *his* fault, *his* bad choice, and *his* responsibility. But he had help. None of us live in a vacuum. When evidence was presented documenting how the tobacco giants had been deceptive in their promotions and claims, people began seeing *them* as part of the problem. We came to understand that we had been tricked. And the courts agreed. Today big tobacco repays the states for health-care costs associated with smoking.

Do parallels exist between tobacco and the processed food industry? Brzezinski quotes Banzshaf further: "They [food companies] are much more worried that this is going to hurt them than tobacco companies ever were. Tobacco companies already wear a very, very black hat. The food companies are reacting to the fact that we are beginning to put a black hat on them."

In 2006, the U.K. banned junk food advertisements during television programming aimed at children. That same year, the European Union regulated that any food making a nutritional claim (such as "low in fat") must also declare on the label if it was high in sugar or salt. Currently the U.S. government is looking into similar ways to educate the public. And that's the key—to educate Joe (and Josephine) Public that there are choices when it comes to eating and choices carry consequences. As more and more people become unhealthy (and health care becomes managed sick care, and managed sick care becomes very expensive), don't be surprised when junk food will eventually be as villainized as cigarettes. It will take time, but it is already beginning to happen. Like cigarettes, it may be gradual and generational. But one thing is for sure: obesity has become a national problem that affects our health and, eventually, your wealth.

Show Me the Money

As a former small business owner I will tell you straight out—*it's all about the money*. While such is an oversimplification—especially since we loved our interaction with customers—at the end of the business day, the bottom line is still the bottom line. Businesses are in business to make money. If they don't, they are out of business. Call it Economics 101.

It's not any different for large food corporations. They, too, are in business to make money. And since salt, sugar, and fat are the staples of processed foods, the question asked of lab-coated food scientists by gray-suited executives in boardrooms across the country is this: how much do we need of each in order to guarantee the maximum return for our investment? In other words, how low can we go and still give the people what they want (taste) and make the investors (Wall Street) happy? Like everything else, it comes down to one thing: profit margin.

It's not any different in the grocery business. Grocery stores are in business to make money, too (for some odd reason, they don't give their stuff away). Go figure. Grocers are in stiff competition to outsell one another and anyone in the grocery business will confirm that.

It's not any different in the restaurant business. National chains along with Mom and Pop establishments are out to make a buck—*yours*. They continue to increase food servings (take off the food and look at the size of the plate), tempt us with fried-up saucy appetizers, and reward us with all-you-can-drink sugar-laced carbonated beverages. Does it work? Let me put it this way: good luck finding a parking place! And if/when you do, they'll hand you a buzzer that will go off in about forty-five minutes. Bon appétit!

Sadly, it costs more to eat healthy. All of which means the obesity issue also involves an economic one. Anyone who has ever shopped "healthy" knows it costs. And for those on a tight budget or families feeding four or five, money plays a significant role when it comes to food choices. That's why it's important to the health of those we love to shop smart, take advantage of local and fresh produce (farmers markets are wonderful!), and get back to the basics of fruits and vegetables. With a little planning and smarter choices, we *can* eat healthier. For example, the next time you eat out at one of those portion-explosion restaurants with plates the size of Cadillac wheel covers, order your favorite dish...and an extra wheel cover. Then split the entrée with your spouse. You can also enjoy the meal while sipping on cool, refreshing, and FREE ice-water with lemon (fruit). Don't be surprised if both your wallet and your waistline are thankful.

What Now?

Overweight people represent the majority of the United States. We didn't get that way by accident. Granted, most are **not** food addicts, but some are. Truthfully, most fall into the category of mindless eaters who have followed the crowd through the drive-thru and into the couch potato rut of overextended waistlines. And while we seek to be sensitive, we do no one any favors by bypassing the issue.

NBC's health correspondent, Dr. Nancy Silverman, believes we need to put the word "fat" back into our vocabulary. Not in an unkind way but in a realistic attempt to help us see the seriousness of the problem. And I would add the same for "addiction." Both are strong words that force accountability, make us look at ourselves, and encourage us to take proactive steps to do better and get healthier. Maybe you need to have that painful conversation with a friend. Maybe you need to have that painful conversation with a parent. Maybe you need to have that painful conversation with...*you.*

On Season 14 of *The Biggest Loser,* a large segment of the show focused on childhood obesity. Sunny Chandrasekar, age 16, had an ongoing struggle with weight-related issues. Working with trainers and nutritionists connected with the program, she learned new eating and exercise habits that changed her life. But the show's biggest moment came when this teenager went home to Rochester, New York, and had a brave and emotional conversation with her overweight mother about the health concerns she had for her. It was a heart-wrenching scene and one impossible to watch without tears. You hurt for the teenager and you hurt for the mother. Yet ultimately it was a conversation that had to be. Sunny, in a moment of incredible maturity well beyond her years, may have saved her mother's life.

The purpose in such a loving intervention is not condemnation (the accused feels self-condemned already). The purpose has a higher motivation: **love.** It's about getting healthier. It's about living longer. It's about being around for your kids and grandkids. It's about offering God and His kingdom-work the best *you* that *you* can be.

You may be in your 30s or 40s, a junk-food junkie, and healthy as a horse (although some horses aren't very healthy). But you won't always be in your 30s and 40s. Double those age numbers and project into the future. What kind of shape will you be in then?

And while we don't have to smoke, we do have to eat. But we don't have to keep eating an overabundance of cake and cookies, chips and snacks, and all those high-calorie processed foods filled with salt, sugar, and fat and loaded with chemicals we can't pronounce. While we don't supersize our bowls of broccoli or carrots, we have no problem supersizing the cheap junk that passes as food. And we keep coming back for more. Do you think we are "hooked?" We may think of them as *happy meals* today, but they may not be so happy years from now. You don't become unhealthy over night. You don't become healthy overnight either. Sadly, many of my fellow baby boomers are waking up today and wishing they had made better choices years ago. It has caught up to them. And it will eventually catch up with you.

It is essential that we get back to a wholesome relationship with food. We must embrace this simple and fundamental change of behavior that realigns us with God's original intent for the human body. Here it is: **we eat to live rather than live to eat.** And because we eat to live, we eat the kind of food that will help us live as healthy and as long as possible.

At some point we have to tell the truth. Political correctness merely skirts the issue and looks the other way. We did that in the 50s and 60s when we buried our heads in our hands and hid beneath our desks. We can't do that any more.

CHAPTER 8

The Biggest Loser

Do you know that those who run in a race all run, but only
one receives the prize? Run in such a way that you may win.
Everyone who competes in the games exercises self-control in all
things. They then do it to receive a perishable wreath, but we an
imperishable. Therefore I run in such a way, as not without aim,
I box in such a way, as not beating the air; but I discipline my body
and make it my slave, so that, after I have preached to others,
I myself will not be disqualified. (1 Corinthians 9:24-27)

The Biggest Loser, NBC's hit reality show, made its debut in October 2004. Ten years later (an eternity in TV-time) it remains a fan favorite. The show features obese individuals and couples competing to see who can lose the most weight. The *biggest loser* is actually the biggest winner and takes home a considerable cash prize in the show's finale. Season 14 even featured a segment on the epidemic of childhood obesity by following three teenagers who struggled with weight issues. Although in the end there is one grand prize winner (alongside one "At Home Winner"—contestants who have been voted off the show, but who are invited to return to see who lost the most weight while at home), in a sense, all of those who participated in the program become winners by losing, too.

Filmed mostly at the King Gillette Ranch near Malibu, California (yes, it is named after the founder of the razor company), the contestants are sequestered from their homes, families, friends, employment, school, etc., while the episodes are filmed. Grouped into three competing teams, each team is assigned a personal trainer who oversees their workouts regiments and offers instruction regarding nutrition. However, it's up to the contestants themselves to perform the workouts and follow the principles they are taught.

Each week culminates with a "weigh-in" to see which team has lost the most. And each week one contestant is "voted" off the show and must leave the Ranch. As the numbers of contestants shrink, the teams are eventually dissolved as they begin to compete individually for the grand prize. In the meantime, millions of viewers tune in each week and find themselves cheering for (or against!) certain ones.

The transformations occurring on the show are extraordinary. To see obese individuals who had given up hope begin to believe in themselves and drop the pounds while often ridding themselves of mental and emotional baggage is indeed encouraging. To that end, the program is especially motivating.

Reality TV or Non-Reality TV?

It is essential to understand that *The Biggest Loser* television program is exactly that—it's *television*. And reality shows are often anything other than...*reality*. Here are some negatives...

First, not everyone can put their life on hold and walk away from their family, homes, jobs, and personal lives for an extended period of time during which they focus entirely on losing weight. That's not real. True reality is what happens every day at home and work in the nuts and bolts of life. In a perfect world where everything we do and eat is monitored, where we have personal trainers, physicians, and dieticians watching our every move, it would be easier to be big losers. But that's not real. Most of us cannot afford to place life on hold.

Second, the results are not that typical. Most healthy weight loss guidelines, doctors, and trainers say that people can lose safely an average of two pounds per week. Yet that hardly makes for dynamite television when viewers would rather see contestants shrieking and screaming because they lost 10 to 20 pounds per week. There is a word for *Biggest*

Loser contestants that lose two pounds per week: *eliminated*. Even during the show's final weeks when weight loss slows to more normal results, contestants are often disappointed. Remember the children's story of the tortoise and the hare? Who won the race? Slow and steady usually wins. Translation: you are more likely to lose the weight and keep it off when you lose gradually and change your lifestyle than when you go to dieting and exercise extremes. We've all known those who have gone crazy with diets and exercise. And what usually happened? Case closed.

Third, it's all about the money. NBC pays its TV trainers mega-bucks to showcase their talents and personalities for the show. And without those electric personalities and often nose-to-nose confrontations and verbal tirades (along with tender moments where trainers morph into psychologists), there would be no show. As a result, advertisers line up to fund the show for the simple reason that people watch. No viewers + no advertisers = no show. Like anything else in the entertainment world, it is ultimately driven by dollars.

Fourth, contestants rely completely on trainers telling them *what* to do, *when* to do it, and *how often*. How nice it would be to have your own personal trainer 24/7—someone to follow you to the gym, to the grocery store, to the office (you know, when co-workers send out for fast-food and you are tempted), and to accompany you to the fridge when a nighttime hunger spell comes calling. Obviously, the trainers didn't literally follow them 24/7, but the cameras did. However, in real-time, there are no cameras. In real-time, a good trainer will train, but not foster a co-dependent relationship.

Fifth, most physical trainers are not therapists. They can help you in ways related to your health and can even give you better tools to believe in what can be accomplished, but most are not psychiatrists or psychologists.

Sixth, TV producers love to create characters and drama. It's why a cross-section of people are chosen in the first place—people whom you love to love and people whom you grow to despise. And by filming continually throughout the week, television can create their own mini-dramas surrounding any one of them.

For example, in season 14, much of the drama surrounded Gina McDonald, a southern lawyer from Birmingham, Alabama. After all, everyone loves to see a good lawyer crash and burn (especially a lawyer with a southern accent). However, Gina didn't crash and burn—she kept on winning, I mean...losing. The drama intensified and the producers undoubtedly loved it. Gina was characterized as the villain and people tuned in each week to watch her for the same reason that many watch NASCAR— hoping for a total meltdown wreck. What they didn't know was that Gina wasn't at all like the person portrayed on the screen. In some ways, she was the opposite. Given the opportunity to meet her in person as Julie and I experienced, you come away wondering: *Is this the same person we just watched last Monday night?*

Given enough film and footage, TV producers can create their own drama stories by cutting and splicing, showing scenes out of sequence, and leaving whatever impression will impact the most viewers. It's not exactly rocket science. I was speaking recently in Pennsylvania and made a comic quip about one of the video producers. She was quick to remind me to be careful because, "I can make you say whatever *I* want you to say." Fortunately she said it with a smile, but I have no doubt she could do exactly that.

Gina McDonald is one of the kindest persons you will ever meet, but you would never know it from watching the program. So, viewer beware. *The Biggest Loser* reality show can easily become more Hollywood than reality.

Biggest Loser Pros

Are there positives about *The Biggest Loser* program? Absolutely. Any time you can teach with a purpose of helping the hurting strive for healthier lifestyles by eating better, exercising, and changing their habits, it is a noble cause. Undoubtedly, many viewers have found motivation to change their own lives by watching *The Biggest Loser*. Good for them. I listed six negatives, so consider six positives:

- **It opens the conversation.** There can be no solution to a problem unless the problem is admitted. *The Biggest Loser* brings the obesity epidemic to the forefront and opens us up to a greater discussion. Ultimately this may be the biggest benefit of all.

- **Success requires accountability.** If the contestants had done well on their own they would have never been chosen for the program in the first place. Personal accountability trainers aside, biggest loser members learn to work together as a team—pulling for and encouraging each other to work harder, exercise longer, and stick to their diet plans. The idea of strength in numbers is Biblical. "Two are better than one because they have a good return for their labor. For if either of them falls, the one will lift up his companion. But woe to the one who falls when there is not another to lift him up" (Eccl.4:9-10). Making a decision to change your life and become health-conscious and proactive with exercise can be daunting if you are alone. But having a friend or support group will provide the extra incentive you need. It's interesting to note that of the four people whose stories we told in chapter one, all of them owed their success to accountability. It works wonders.

- **Surround yourself with positive people.** The negative nay-sayers on *The Biggest Loser* don't last (the remaining contestants are actually strengthened by the absence of these excuse-makers). Negative people will drain any motivation you have to change—regardless of the area that needs changing. One of the biggest themes from the program is to help each contestant change their own negative thinking in ways they had not previously considered. Sadly, we are often our own worst enemy when it comes to self-talk. As each show progresses you can see the positive brain-training kick in. Soon "I can't" becomes "I can!" and eventually "I will!"—as the remaining contestants come to believe in themselves.

- **It takes hard work and total dedication.** One of my favorite moments is when the trainers meet the contestants outside the gym on the first day of workouts. In season 14, trainers Bob Harper, Jillian Michaels, and Dolvett Quince laughed at the ladies who had taken the time to put on their makeup (and why not, they were going on television). However, sweat and makeup don't mix. Exercise is not easy (if it was, it wouldn't do any good). It's the very reason why thousands of people say they want to lose weight and get into better physical condition, but few are those who pay the price or sacrifice to see results. Half-hearted efforts go nowhere. Give these folks the credit due—they work hard.

- **It's essential to have some fun.** *The Biggest Loser* presents new and different challenges each week. It's actually fun to watch teams compete in challenges ranging from running escalators to crossing a ravine on a zip-line; from digging for arrows in a sand dune to holding team members' hands while crossing a high wire. The one thing you cannot say about *The Biggest Loser* is that the challenges/workouts are boring. Boring will kill any exercise routine. So undo the routine. Remember Michelle from chapter one? Some days she works out at sunrise with her group at Boot Camp and some days she works out—*with her kids at the playground.* If variety is the spice of life, mix it up and have some fun.

- **Finish what you start.** One of the biggest and best moments on *The Biggest Loser* is when the contestants who were voted off and were sent home get to return and compete at a final weigh-in for the "At Home" prize. It is amazing to see the transformation—of both body and mind (you can't have one without the other). Regardless of the season you watch, the biggest losers are always those who were consistent and kept the end in focus. They made a life-change—even after they returned home. And if they can do it, so can you.

The Biggest Loser's Biggest Con

My biggest gripe with the show isn't with the show at all (with a few exceptions—including foul-mouthed trainers who, for whatever reason, spew unnecessary profanities and with producers who think such garbage is necessary), but with the people who, season after season, keep "trying out" while waiting to be chosen. It's as if their success at life-change depends upon their being on *The Biggest Loser.* That's sad. And telling. Is the prerequisite for finding your own personal turning point to be chosen for a television reality show? Apparently to some it is. One hopeful contestant-to-be is quoted as saying,

"I've tried three times to get on The Biggest Loser. I'm sixty and need to get this weight off."

Houston, we've got a problem.

If this lady is sixty, obese, and a *Biggest Loser* groupie, she needs to get a life by taking charge of her own. Her time is running out and so is her health. Tragically, she is one of many.

Let's cut to the chase. Those chosen on *The Biggest Loser* are not celebrities. They are overweight people who have allowed themselves to become that way by the choices they made in regard to food and exercise. Eventually those bad choices caught up with them. But give them credit for trying... which is more than many are willing to do. And to those who learned and tasted success, I adjure you to use the new you as a precious gift from God and give back. *Give back* to others who need your encouragement. *Give back* to those who have given up. *Give back* at every opportunity to touch a hurting life. *Give back.*

There are pros and cons to most everything. The underlying themes of *The Biggest Loser* are sound: eat real food in reasonable amounts, exercise consistently, drink water, and surround yourself with positive people who will encourage your quest and, at the same time, provide a measure of accountability. Tuning into the show can be both informational and motivational. It's essential, however, that you separate fact from fiction, reality from non-reality television.

The Biggest Loser's Gina McDonald— 6 Tips On How to Lose Weight At Home
from *Girl Get Strong* Magazine
(reprinted with permission of the editor)

Losing it at home was incredibly hard. I lost 29 pounds during the 8 weeks at home and worked harder than any time I spent on the Ranch. My six tips are:

1. Believe you can make changes in your daily life that will impact the remainder of your life in a very positive way. For me, realizing that I could do this at home and having faith and belief in the process changed everything for me. Remember that sometimes our body does not respond as quickly as we want it to. Some weeks at home I lost zero pounds, but worked harder than ever and was on point with diet. Then the next week: Bam! I had to maintain my belief in the process day-to-day.

2. Organize. I became very orderly while training at home and have maintained that order since the finale. To not organize leads to chaos and with chaos we lose control of the things that are within our control. I take steps every night to plan and organize my day. What I am wearing to work out, food choices, errands, etc.

3. Sleep. Sleep is critical for our bodies and minds. I made sure that I got 8-10 hours of rest time each day.

4. Starve no more! You have to eat to lose weight. Eating lean protein balanced with fat and carbohydrates worked for me.

5. Monitor. I monitored every aspect of my day using my BodyMedia armband. Knowing your calorie burn each day, sleep patterns, and logging your meals takes all the guesswork out of your day.

6. Exercise. I exercised a lot during my time at home, but now I do cardio one hour a day and body weight and strength conditioning for thirty minutes.

As a lawyer and law firm owner, 47-year-old Gina McDonald is very accomplished in her professional life. Getting control of her lifelong struggle with weight has proved to be a greater challenge. The Memphis, Tennessee native grew up in Vicksburg, Mississippi, the middle child of three children and got a business degree from Northwest Louisiana University and a law degree from Birmingham School of Law in Alabama. She got to a healthy weight when she started practicing law, but she began getting heavier after a divorce in 2002 left her a single mother of two young children. Poor eating habits, lack of exercise, and the stress of divorce and dealing with emotional issues were all contributing factors. Now 245 pounds, with weight-related health issues that have included sleep apnea, high cholesterol, diabetes and hypothyroidism, Gina wants to finally become fit and healthy. She looks forward to running a marathon, playing golf with her husband, having the energy to work longer days and just enjoy life. "My whole life I have dreamed of being fit and healthy," she says. "Now I have the courage, desire, dedication and opportunity to finally make my dreams come true."

And she did.

Gina weighed 245 pounds when she found her turning point. She went on to lose 132 pounds and freely admits she is a work in progress. She enjoys living life out loud and especially overjoyed living without type 2 diabetes. Julie and I count her as a friend and have enjoyed watching her journey. She credits her trainers on *The Biggest Loser* and her at-home trainer, Carter Hays. Above all, she credits the Lord.

Gina regularly puts out encouraging ideas and motivational thoughts via Facebook. Connect with her using that medium. She and other former contestants on *The Biggest Loser* give back by participating in various walks and runs benefiting worthy causes. You will find her to be engaging, gracious, and kind. And...a positive encourager in your own journey toward better health.

Note: Contestants on The Biggest Loser *sign a contractual agreement not to disclose particular elements of the program or use the program in ways that would benefit them financially (e.g., a tell-all book). As a result, no contestant was interviewed for this book. The information contained in this chapter represents my own opinions resulting from personal observations.*

CHAPTER 9

Eat Your Fruits and Vegetables, and...Work on That Attitude

Beloved, I pray that in all respects you may prosper
and be in good health, just as your soul prospers. (3 John 2)

The Garden of Eden was exactly that—a garden. Last time I checked, gardens grow fruits and vegetables. That hasn't changed since the beginning of time. When the spies of Old Testament Israel returned from their reconnaissance mission (Numbers 13), they "cut down a cluster of grapes...with some of the pomegranates and figs" (v.23). They returned to the people and "showed them the fruit of the land" (v.26). When God spoke of His love for His people, He spoke of them as "the apple of His eye" (Zechariah 2:8). When a young maiden described her beloved, she compared him to "an apple tree among the trees of the forest" (Song of Solomon 2:3). A fitting remark made at an appropriate time is compared poetically to "apples of gold in settings of silver" (Proverbs 25:11).

Have you ever looked at the ingredient list on the side of an apple? No you haven't because *there is no ingredient list on the side of an apple*. If one did exist, it would say: This apple contains...*apple*. Imagine that. If you don't believe that, look at the ingredient list on the side of a tomato. Or spinach. The great thing about God's "reproducing after its kind" meal plan is that you can march out to the garden (or go to your local Farmer's Market like we do), load up, wash off, and eat. Of course, if you're like me and prefer your green beans cooked rather than crunchy, steam away and then eat. Anyway, it's not that complicated.

Fruits and vegetables...The key to maximizing your effectiveness before God is to live as healthy as you can. And that means fruits and vegetables rather than fast and processed foods. Fruits and veggies provide antioxidants to build healthy cells (hopefully you were there the day they taught you this in Health 101). And healthy cells just happen to be your body's front-line defense against oxidative stress. That's why you need those antioxidants. They are the good that neutralizes the bad. In other words, if you don't eat your fruits and vegetables, the body will give way to disease and premature aging. And you don't want that.

Okay, let's cut to the chase. We've all been hearing this same-song-second-verse refrain since we were kids. "Eat your vegetables, dear, so you can grow up healthy and strong." What most of us learned to do early on was the old divide and conquer trick—push the peas and carrots around on our plate to make it look like we actually ate them (or better yet, feed them secretly to the dog lurking beneath the table). Vegetables, after all, were tasteless and mushy and made you think of hospital or prison food (or at least the middle school cafeteria, which seemed like prison).

The adults in our lives obsessed about us eating our vegetables. The conversation usually connected our hesitancy with a speech about little boys and girls in China who would love to eat our vegetables—if they only had them. Apparently the whole idea of farm-produce export hadn't occurred to our parents.

Our parents, however, were right (although the China motivation may have been skewed). Hopefully we have caught up to the nutritional learning curve. By the looks of things, however, I have my doubts.

The experts in the medical field are unanimous when it comes to connecting fruit and vegetables with healthier living. Almost daily, another piece of research comes to light that heralds the risk-reducing power of our dietary choices and the healthy benefits of eating more fruits and vegetables.

Sadly, America seems fixated on over-the-counter vitamins as a quick and easy alternative. It really isn't. Julie explains,

> First of all, the vitamin pill you buy is man-made. What happens is a process wherein you remove from fruits andvegetables a particular component you want and leave the others. Research is learning, however, that the vitamin you extracted worked best in harmony with all the other minerals and nutrients that were in that fruit or veggie naturally. It now loses its synergy. The bioavailability of a fruit or vegetable is received by the body and put to work much quicker than a man-made product on the shelf. That's why getting real fruits and vegetables give your body what it craves. And since fruits and vegetables were created by God specifically for your body, it automatically knows what to do with it.

That's another way of saying the same thing: eat your fruits and vegetables. We need the real deal. It makes sense. The thousands of nutrients God put in real food work together in ways that science is just beginning to understand and that no man-made vitamin or synthetic pill will replace.

The message is clear: we need more whole food nutrition in our daily food intake. It's the one thing everyone agrees we can do to improve our health and reduce the risk of disease. Something tells me you already knew that. Like in many things, however, knowledge isn't our problem.

Remember Jared?

Jared Fogle was so fat he had trouble squeezing into some of the classroom seats at Indiana University. He would ride the 45-minute shuttle bus to class rather than walk the five minutes from his dorm. He drank as many as 15 cans of soda a day and had a diet that consisted mainly of junk food: cheeseburgers, fries, soft drinks, and desserts. He tipped the scales at 425 pounds (the equivalent weight of an adult bear). He had sleep apnea because the fat around his neck obstructed his windpipe. His life was a mess.

In the spring of 1998, Jared walked into a Subway restaurant and found his *turning point*. He made the decision to reduce his calorie consumption from 10,000 to 2,000. His no-nonsense solution was to order a 6-inch turkey sub with no cheese, no mayo, veggies and spicy mustard. He added a small bag of baked chips. He drank water. For supper he returned and ordered a foot-long veggie sub and baked chips. He drank water. He began to lose weight. His father, a physician, encouraged him to add exercise to his new eating habits. Jared stopped riding the shuttle-bus and began walking to class. In three months he was down 94 pounds (eventually he lost a total of 245 pounds). Today Jared is known mainly as "The Subway Guy."

You've probably seen him on commercials showing off his 58" waistline pants as a reminder of what used to be. In 2010 he trained, ran, and completed the New York City Marathon. According to an article in *USA Today* (February 23, 2013, by Bruce Horovitz), Jared cried when he crossed the finish line.

What makes Jared Fogle a hero to so many is that he is so real. He comes across as a nerdy, bespectacled college kid who decided to make a proactive change. His message is unmistakably clear: *If I can do this, so can you.*

In the *USA Today* article cited above, Jared gives six common-sense tips to help others. They are:

1. Watch portion sizes carefully.

2. Eat lots of fruits and veggies.

3. Drink lots of water.

4. Exercise every day.

5. Ask for all sauces and dressings on the side (put them on yourself, sparingly).

6. Don't let a bad day, or week, or month change your diet plans.

Did you happen to catch #2? It's not rocket science.

Stuff You Need to Know

Fruits and vegetables are the cornerstone to a healthy diet. Not only are they full of all those vitamins and minerals your body needs, but also full of water and fiber. The water and fiber are what gives you the "full" feeling that can make a positive contribution to weight loss. That's common sense, too. If your brain is sending you the "Whoa!" signal, you are less likely to overindulge. Livestrong.com suggests…

As a general rule of thumb, the darker or more colorful a fruit or vegetable is, the higher it will be in vitamins, minerals, and antioxidants. Red strawberries, dark green kale, and bright yellow squash are all bursting with nutrients for a healthy life. Vitamins and minerals help your body function, keeping your heart pumping regularly, your skin clear and soft and your vision crisp and clear, and antioxidants boost your immunity, helping your body fight off everything from the common cold to cancer. Choose a variety of fruits and vegetables in a rainbow of colors for a wide selection of vitamins, minerals, and antioxidants.

Hey, that's what my mom said. Well, maybe not exactly. But I do remember something about carrots and rabbits that never wear glasses.

And the fiber...the fiber works to fight off heart disease since the fiber pushes cholesterol through your pipes, preventing it from being absorbed. Think of it as nature's scrub brush keeping your intestines sparkling. And, besides that, it keeps the train running on time. Enough said.

Okay, here's the scoop (or at least the cup). One cup of fruits or vegetables counts as one serving. Got it? Dieticians recommend eating five to nine servings of fruits *and* vegetables every day. I know what you're thinking because I'm thinking it, too. Five to nine servings...*Really?* The truth is, I don't know anyone who does that consistently. Do you? Reports show only 7% of children and adolescents actually consume the recommended daily amount. I'm going out on a limb here, but my guess is that only 7% of their mommies and daddies do, too. But it's good to have a goal, and that's the goal. Consider these top ten ways to improve on the illness-fighting, age-delaying fruits and vegetables:

- Shop the outside isles of the supermarket where they keep the good stuff.

- Keep fresh fruit close and where it can be seen as a snack substitute.

- Cut up carrots, broccoli, and other fresh vegetables and keep them in a sealed container in the fridge where they can be eaten whenever you want them (keep hummus or salsa handy for dipping).

- Keep apples in a bowl on the counter.

- Eat grilled salads for lunch (dressing on the side).

- Eat tossed salads as a side for supper (lots of color).

- Eat vegetable-heavy soups, stews, and stir-fry.

- Eat cereal with added blueberries, bananas, or strawberries (not the pre-packaged processed stuff, but the kind you buy and cut up).

- Eat fruit for dessert.

- Enjoy an occasional single scoop of ice cream (scoop, as in the size of a serving spoon—not scoop, as in the size of a front end loader) and load it up with bits of fruit (blueberries, bananas, peaches, strawberries, etc.).

- Shop your local farmer's market for the freshest produce.

Oops, that's eleven, so consider the last as one to "grow on." Eat healthier—live healthier—enjoy life longer. If you can develop good eating habits (eat more of the good stuff and less of the bad stuff) in your earlier years, your body will pay you dividends in your latter ones. "An apple a day..."

Broccoli... Yuk!
Broccoli... Yep!

If any of you knew me back when...you are snickering about now. I applauded years ago when President George H. W. Bush (#41) laid down the law in the Oval Office. He said, "I do not like broccoli, and I haven't liked it since I was a little kid and my mother made me eat it. And I'm President of the United States, and I'm not going to eat any more broccoli. Now look, this is the last statement I'm going to have on broccoli. There are truckloads of broccoli at this very minute descending on Washington. My family is divided. For the broccoli vote out there, Barbara loves broccoli. She has tried to make me eat it. She eats it all the time herself. So she can go out and meet the caravan of broccoli that's coming in..." I love decisiveness in a leader.

I have no clue if the president ever learned to like broccoli. Somewhere along the way, however, *I* did. I'm not crazy for a whole big pile of it, but in the right proportions and included in a Chinese stir fry or with some seasoning or in salads, I'm a "go." I know. It blows your mind.

There are still some vegetables I'm not crazy about, but let's say I have learned to expand my palate (not plate—*palate*). Julie and I enjoy eating lunch out at places like Jason's Deli or Ruby Tuesday's because of their great salad bars where you can load up on all the rainbow vegetables you want to eat. FYI: Smothering them with a fatty dressing misses the point. Be smart. We've learned to get an extra plate or bowl for the dressing and just "dip" as needed. And most fast food places offer some great salads— many with grilled chicken. Once again, watch the dressing ("watch," as in "not eat"—or eat a very small amount).

So much of this comes down to common sense. You know what's good for you, and you know what's not good for you. It's easy to eat more fruits and vegetables, but…it's even easier not to. Like anything else, you have to be proactive in your decision making. *Think! Think! Think!* As in, *think* about what goes on your fork.

Fuel for Thought

About now I need an illustration that a warm-bloodied American male can grab onto. Here goes. Gasoline is the fuel that provides the energy to power your car. We fill up and thus provide our engine with the "spark" it needs until the "Low Fuel" light comes on again. Come to think of it, it's a lot like fuel for another mode of transportation: our body. We fill up at the table and find the "spark" to "live, move, and have our being" until the dashboard of our brain lights up and says it's time to refuel. Sometimes we use premium-grade fuel and sometimes we buy the cheaper stuff that holds us over to the next refueling station. Funny thing about us humans, we often provide better fuel for our cars than for our bodies. I wonder what would happen if a gas station advertised—"Our gas isn't as good as theirs, but it's a lot cheaper!" No one would put cheap, junky gas in their car. Why not? Because we know that doing so will cost us more money in the long run when it comes to repairs. (This is where the "duh" light should come on).

However, here's the kicker. We don't change the oil—that golden fluid that keeps the engine running smoothly and lasting longer. Why is it that some engines last 50,000 miles while others last 200,000 miles? Simple. Engine life expectancy is tied to changing the oil. And when it comes to our marvelous bodies, what is the oil that keeps us running smoother and longer?

Ahem...*fruits and vegetables.*

But who has time to eat them? And all those servings? It's a whole lot easier to grab a Pop Tart as you head out the door in the morning rush, a burger for lunch, and finally pizza for supper. Of course, we're made to feel better if it's a "cherry" Pop Tart ("It does have fruit, right?" Uh, read the label...), and we throw a slice of tomato on the burger, and maybe pepperoni on the pizza (note: pepperoni isn't a vegetable). Sure, the low-fuel light goes off and we feel full, but the oil in our engine is slowly clogging up. We are very meticulous about changing the oil in our cars every three to five thousand miles, but what about the circulation fluids in our body engines? That seems backward to me.

By the way, if you think auto mechanics charge an arm and a leg for a new engine, you haven't priced doctors lately.

Diet is a Four-Letter Word (It's Also a Noun)

It's time for a little English 101...

The word "diet" should be a noun, as in: "His diet is rich in fruits and vegetables," rather than a verb: "I need to go on a diet." The problem with *diet* as a verb is that it signifies action (what verbs do) that is temporary at best (what cheap verbs do). Used in this way, it signifies something negative and is associated with the synonymous "starving" or "not eating." It's why "verb diets" don't work. On the other hand, "noun diets" do work because they involve a change in one's nutritional discipline. In other words, rather than a temporary quick fix, noun diets become a lifestyle.

Most verb diets don't work because they don't really change anything. We get gung-ho about the latest fad that cuts out this or eliminates that, but it doesn't last. Sure, simply restricting calories will cause you to lose weight, but it will also cause you to get hungry. Very hungry! A healthier (and smarter!) choice is to go on a noun diet—to make the lifestyle choice that combines healthy eating with exercise. "Diet" should *name* the action, not *be* the action! It's not about starving the body for food but fueling it with the right food. It has to be a lifestyle change.

Julie has some thoughts...

I hate the word "diet." It is a four-letter word that I am ridding from my vocabulary! First of all when you start using the word diet, it usually goes like this... "Well, I have to start dieting again." Or, "No thank you, I'm on a diet." That type of talk is self-defeating. It immediately puts you in a sour mood as if you are punishing yourself for bad behavior. And while you and I have made our share of poor choices, changing directions in your life (finding your "turning point") must be done with positive outlooks and positive talk.

If you are like me, you have "yo-yoed" with food choices, trying to find your place and discover who you are. And there is a strong desire to find peace in all of that, to find acceptance and be pleased with the outcome. You give attention to every new "weight loss program" out there and try it, hoping to find the "magic" spell that you knew was all there all along. You were just waiting for it to be discovered!

But there is no magic spell. There is no quick fix. There is "nothing new under the sun." What happens with your body and with your mind must come from within you. Certainly it is good to be held accountable when working to make changes in your life, but at the end of the day...it all comes back to you.

It is my opinion that in order to make your life change for the better in anything you do, you must learn to think through all your decisions. I know, it can be a hassle. It would be so much easier to just skip through life and do whatever you want, but remember this is not magical—this is life. It has taken years for me to learn this. I wanted to skip! But when I realized all those other ways weren't working to keep me healthy, I realized my journey and my participation in it was critical.

What held me back in making the best choices for my life...was *me.* I let others decide for me by doing what they did. If they made poor food choices, so did I. If they could eat a big piece of chocolate cake or a plateful of chips or that thick ice cream with all those candies in it, then so could I. This is not saying you couldn't ever have cake or chips or ice cream. What it is saying is that you have to think through what you are going to consume and ask: Is it worth it? I can't tell you how many times I have eaten something in the excitement of the moment—and yes, it can be exciting—to then realize I had made a big mistake. I would ask myself, "Why did you do that?" In other words, did I even think?

DIET
Did
I
Even
Think

And, of course, I could always talk myself out of exercising. "You mean I am supposed to sweat? What about my hair?" Do you see the "yo-yo" now?

Your body craves good food if you give it good food. And by good food, I mean food that will nourish your body toward health and long living. It is tempting to be depressed about the way you "used" to be. But don't go there. Your time is NOW! Your "turning point" is NOW! Make the decision today that you are no longer going to let others decide what you put in your body. YOU are in control of this. The body you have depends on you to take care of it, so give it what it needs to function at its best. Sometimes we think our bodies are best showcased bronzed and buffed. But what is happening on the inside? Skipped meals and starving attitudes destroy the function of this God-created machine that longs for movement and energy. We want the latest upgrades for our houses: a man-made shelter. But we give our "God-made" shelter…junk.

You are worth so much more than junk. You deserve the upgrade, which actually is very simple. Fruits, vegetables, lean protein and water. You will have to think about it though. Think about what is best for you. In time, it will come naturally to make better choices. I never thought I would miss a power walk or an exercise challenge that I knew I couldn't do (thank you, Carter Hays)!

You will know when your turning point is real. Nothing holds you back from making best choices. And when someone asks if you are "dieting," you say: "No, I am making better choices for me." And you will smile to yourself. In fact...you might be tempted to start skipping!

Reality Check

I don't eat five to nine servings of fruits and vegetables every day either. I know some who have tried to do so by "juicing" (no, I'm not talking about steroids and baseball), but that ends up being time consuming and costly. It's also nigh to impossible when you're traveling. So, what's a man, woman, or child to do?

We made the decision to "juice" another way. Our family takes Juice Plus+ which has been scientifically studied and is the most researched nutritional product in the world. It is not a vitamin. It is whole food nutrition from a variety of fruits and vegetables. In fact, it has twenty-six. These are juiced and concentrated into powders. We take them each day in order to experience the benefit from real fruits and vegetables. So, when someone asks if I eat the recommended five to nine daily servings of fruits and vegetables, my literal answer is, "No. In fact, I eat *more*—as in twenty-six!" From the orchard I get: apple, orange, pineapple, cranberry, papaya, peach, and cherry. From the garden I get: carrot, parsley, beet, kale, broccoli, cabbage, spinach, tomato, oat bran, and brown rice bran. And from the vineyard I get: grape, blueberry, cranberry, blackberry, bilberry, raspberry, red currant, black currant, and elderberry. They come in capsules or gummy chewables. And get this: our grandkids love 'em! Whoa. Imagine that. (FYI: Juice Plus+ has an excellent program to help children get their fruits and vegetables free. I like free.)

I'm not trying to sell you anything. There is information in the back of the book if you would like to know more. And if you're prone to skepticism, so was I.

Two years ago, I was a severe asthmatic living on inhalers and steroids. It wasn't cheap, and the side effects weren't fun. Today I am on zero meds! In 2010, Julie was diagnosed with macular degeneration and began a series of eye injections (twelve, to be specific) to slow down this dreaded disease. Since adding Juice Plus+ to her daily regimen, the physicians at Vanderbilt

Eye Institute have been amazed. Her vision has stabilized. We walked away relieved and thankful to the Lord for what He has provided.

I'm more inclined to put stock in what has worked for me. That's ditto for her—except that as a medical professional she is also inclined to put stock in clinical studies. Regardless, we have experienced positive results firsthand.

Don't take my word for it.

> "Products such as Juice Plus+, currently under study in my lab, take all the nutrients from plant foods and concentrate them into capsules for those who simply can't or won't eat the recommended servings (that's most Americans!). Unlike multivitamins which take nutrients out of context and repackage them, whole food supplements maintain the natural array and concentration of nutrients—thousands of them—found in the food themselves. It may be that nutrients only work as they should in concert, like the various instruments in a symphony."

**David Katz, M.D., Yale University Research Prevention Center
Article in the *Huffington Post***

> "Medical colleagues often ask me why I feel so strongly about recommending Juice Plus+. I tell them I think it would be unethical of me not to recommend it, knowing what I know about the product and the science behind it. People don't eat as well as they should, and I'm no exception. That's why I've taken Juice Plus+ every day for more than 15 years."

**Richard DuBois, M.D., Former President Georgia Society of
Internal Medicine, President of the Medical Association of Atlanta**

> "Juice Plus+ is the only daily supplement I take. Do your children get sick all the time? Do you frequently feel tired and run down? Is it nearly impossible to get your children to eat fruits and vegetables? Are you lacking the recommended servings of fruits and vegetables each day? If the answer to any of these is yes, then Juice Plus is extremely important to you and your family."

**Dr. William Sears, Pediatrician
San Clemente, California**

"I believe Juice Plus+ to be the single source to bridge the gap between what we should eat and what we *do* eat. That's why I take it daily."

Carter Hays, Personal Trainer and Author

Do your own research. I know I feel good (literally!) when I get all those fruits, vegetables, and berries. By the way, have you had your kale today? Spinach? Bilberry? I have. Come to think of it, I've even had my broccoli...

A Disease?

The debate rages as to whether obesity should be labeled a "disease." The American Medical Association recently announced that it will recognize obesity as a disease requiring medical treatment and prevention. My guess is that such a move is motivated more by money than anything else. If obesity is labeled a "disease," then insurance companies will be forced to pay for treatments. All of which means, there is no free lunch (regardless of its nutritional quality). Someone will have to foot the bill as premiums increase with the extra burden. And don't be surprised if that someone is...*you.*

In a nation where it is culturally acceptable to cast blame, shift the burden of responsibility, and expect the government to solve our problems, we are made to feel better if our poor health is not our fault (disease) and someone else's problem (they pay for it). True, some health-related issues are genetic, and I understand metabolism dysfunction. On the other hand, in a nation where eating junk and processed foods have become the national pastime, it can't all fall at the feet of genetics and metabolism.

At the end of the day and at the end of our lives, we each have choices to make regarding our health. And much of our health or lack thereof can be traced to our eating, exercise, and attitude. No one forces you to eat junk and live a sedentary life. On the other hand, no one forces you to get fit and healthy. But as with all choices, there are consequences.

Our problem is not so much "how to" as "want to." Do you want to live healthy and stay productive? Consider a quote from Dr. Carol Watson. Dr. Watson has a double doctorate as a Nutritional Counselor and Doctor of Naturopathy and practices in the Indianapolis area. She makes you think...

If life was about "how to's" we would all be skinny, rich, and happy, right? But there's so much more to it than "the doing." The only way we will ever understand ourselves regardless of the issue—diet, relationships, finances, business—is to become aware of what we are thinking so we can change our results. This is referred to as T-E-A (Thoughts-Emotions-Actions). Change our thoughts and our emotions change, which then creates different actions/behaviors for improved results. It's our thoughts that dictate what we do.

We think 40,000 thoughts per day and 85% of them are the same thoughts over and over. Thoughts like, "I'm not good enough," or "I'm not pretty enough," or "I'm not smart enough," or "I'm not deserving of the love of others." But we so desperately want to change so we try to alter our behavior (or actions) and when that doesn't work, we get frustrated and stuck. This becomes a vicious cycle until we become aware of our thoughts and untwist the lies we have been telling ourselves for years.

Experts estimate that our core beliefs are in place by the time we are about seven years old. The two primary core beliefs are: (1) I'm not worthy (I'm not good enough, so why bother?), or (2) I'm not capable (I've failed in the past, so why try again?). Both are self-defeating. So, since our subconscious mind is what is driving our thoughts, one way to break the pattern of lies is to go to our prayer closet and "be still and know that He is God" (Psalm 46:10). It takes practice and intention to quiet our minds and observe our thoughts; I challenge you to give it a try.

The more I view life from the Christian perspective (who I am and who God created me to be), the more I learn to accept and love myself as the unique and beautiful woman God created in His image. The end result then is that, as I love and accept myself, the opinions of others hold less weight. I like to frame it this way—"What you think of me is none of my business!"

She is right. Change starts at the top—as in the way *you* think. Living the same old way will only give you the same old results. In other words, if nothing changes, nothing changes. Are you ready for a turning point? Then you need to do two things: (1) eat right (lots of fruits and vegetables...*farm-acy* beats *pharm-acy* any day of the week!), and (2) work on your attitude.

The latter involves a whole other chapter.

CHAPTER 10

The Verse That Will Change Your Life

Whatever is true,
Whatever is honorable,
Whatever is right,
Whatever is pure,
Whatever is lovely,
Whatever is of good repute,
If there is any excellence and if anything worthy of praise,
Dwell on these things.
(Philippians 4:8)

How important is your thinking? Let me guess—you're thinking: *Well, I've never given it much thought...* Exactly. If you are what you eat (and you are), more importantly, *you are what you think.* "For as he thinks within himself, so is he" (Proverbs 23:7). What you choose to think about is critical to your self-esteem and success regardless of the battle you're facing.

Most are oblivious when it comes to their habitual thought patterns. Yet, it's either or. *Either* you are motivated to think God-honoring thoughts (seeing yourself as He sees you), *or* you are motivated to think thoughts from, let's say, lesser elevations. True, much of what goes on in life you cannot control. You cannot control the weather, traffic jams, and what others do and say. Yet you have 100% control over what kind of thoughts you allow to roll around between your ears.

What does this have to do with living a healthier life? Everything. You cannot be healthy and happy until you embrace the 4:8 truths.

The Fix Is in...*the Mind*

The turning point for positive change must begin some place. And that "some place" is the four-pound mass of muscle (if you want to get technical, it's an organ), tucked away behind your eyes and carefully protected by the bone of your skull. Paul said, "And do not be conformed to this world, but be transformed **by the renewing of your mind**, so that you may prove what the will of God is..." (Romans 12:2—emphasis mine). Thus, God's child is challenged to step away from the world and live differently. And that difference begins with the way you choose to think.

Note three axioms about your thoughts. **(1) There is a direct relationship between your thoughts and the degree to which you enjoy life.** That is why the sky-is-always-falling drama king or queen isn't exactly the most pleasant person to be around. Have you noticed? **(2) There is a direct relationship between your thoughts and the atmosphere in your marriage and home life.** Negative thinking accentuates the faults of your spouse and children by magnifying them to unrealistic proportions. As a result, minor annoyances become major big deals because we choose to dwell on them rather than see the bigger picture. **(3) There is a direct relationship between your thoughts and how well you interact with others.** Take Bob, for example. If Bob has a problem with Mary and Bob has a problem with Jim and Bob has a problem with John, and Sarah, and Chris—maybe...the...problem...is...*Bob*. The bottom line is this: the way we think determines the course of our life. Don't take my word for it.

> Watch over your heart with all diligence, for from it flow the springs of life. (Proverbs 4:23)

The heart of which Solomon speaks is not the physical one that beats behind your breast. It is the heart that is the seat of your thinking—i.e., your mind.

Contrary to popular belief, we are not limited by our past nor are we imprisoned by our present circumstances. I don't know anyone who has had a guilt-free past or whose present situation is 100% wonderful. So then, if we are not limited by our past or present, then what limits us? Our self-talk. It's the junk-stuff we keep telling ourselves and the junk-stuff we keep believing.

Paul said it is time we discipline our minds to "dwell" on (some translations render it "ponder") "these things." What things? God things. Good things. Things that are true (as opposed to rumor or "What if..."), noble, just, pure, lovely, excellent, etc. Think (there's that word!) how we would impact the people around us in a much better way if we only would flesh out the principles of this passage. Jesus said, "Let your light shine before men in such a way that they may see your good works, and glorify your Father who is in heaven" (Matt.5:16). Glorifying God begins with a life of good works, and good works begin with...good thoughts.

Poor, Poor, Pitiful Paul

If anyone was ever justified in being negative, it was the apostle Paul. Unfairly accused by his adversaries, confined in prison, and facing the sentence of death, Paul writes the letter to the Philippians with a woe-is-me disposition of despair... *"My life is terrible... You don't know how hard I have it... The food here is awful... The guards are mean... It's too cold... I'm not free to come and go like you are..."* Truthfully, that sounds more like A. A. Milne's character, Eeyore, on Winnie-the-Pooh. I know a few Eeyores, and my guess is that you do, too.

Paul chose the opposite mindset. He made a deliberate and proactive decision to discipline his mind so that his thoughts would be God-honoring. And why? Because his thoughts were a reflection of his faith. And...so are yours.

It was no easier for him than it is for you. A few verses later he admits his struggle. He writes, "I have learned to be content in whatever circumstances I am" (v.11). His mindset of contentment and praise-worthy thinking did not come naturally. It was something he had to learn and grow into. It's not natural for you either (or me). But if he could do it, we can, too.

Time for a Mental Upgrade

My family makes fun of me because I am about two decades behind when it comes to technology. By the time I get used to something, it's out of date. I have a Texas friend who laughs at me and says, "Adams' idea of an upgrade is to go to the office supply store and get a new legal pad!" Sadly, that's close to accurate.

Take my phone (my kids say you should—as in, *take it and throw it away!*). Okay, I have a flip phone (remember, the first step in solving a problem is admitting you have one). My flip phone will do two things with which I am comfortable: I can call others and others can call me. I don't text and drive, because...well, I don't text at all. Or rarely—and certainly not well. Last week I left my phone in the cubicle at the fitness center where my wife and I go each week. I went back the next day and there it was, exactly where I left it. I told my son that such was proof that most people are good and honest. He shrugged and sighed, "Dad," he said, "Your phone wasn't stolen because NO ONE WOULD WANT IT!" Okay, I get it. Sort of.

At some point I will need to *upgrade* my phone. At some point, all of us will need to *upgrade* our thinking. And that's what Philippians 4:8 says. *Upgrade your thinking!*

Like the old song, "Looking for love in all the wrong places..." we're looking for joy and peace in all the wrong places. The same writer challenges us in 1 Thessalonians 5:16-18 to commit ourselves to two things: (1) rejoice always, and (2) give thanks about everything. But how can I "rejoice always" if my life isn't always great? And how can I "give thanks" if I am surrounded by circumstances for which I am not thankful? Good questions.

Here is the answer.

Upgrading to become a Philippians 4:8 thinker (a "rejoice always" and "thankful" thinker) doesn't mean that your life is 100% fantastic. I don't know anyone's that is. Paul's wasn't. Yet in spite of life's hardships and hurts, you (like him) can enthusiastically wrap your arms around the living God and stand emphatically upon His promises. Isn't that the essence of faith? "And without faith it is impossible to please Him, for he who comes to God must believe that He is and that He is a rewarder of those who seek Him" (Hebrews 11:6). He doesn't say that without faith it is highly unlikely or improbable to please Him; He says it is impossible.

Here it is: your joy (or lack thereof) is an outward sign of your inside faith. It is indicative of what's going on inside your head. One of the songs little children love to sing goes like this, "I've got the joy, joy, joy, joy down in my heart. Where? Down in my heart…" And Solomon reminds us that if the joy's in your heart (your faith is firmly set in your mind), it will show up on your face. "A joyful heart makes a cheerful face" (Proverbs 15:13).

This has nothing to do with personality. Yes, some people are naturally more outgoing than others who may be reflective and quiet. This is about faith and a way of thinking/acting that says, "I may not understand everything that is happening or know the outcome or even know why, but I trust God with every ounce of my being." Can you trust Him even in the absence of knowing the answer to the "why" question? If you can't, then I fail to grasp the significance of the Job and Joseph stories in Scripture. Or the story of the imprisoned Paul.

If you would upgrade your joy, you would be a lot more fun to be around. Your marriage would be better. Your relationship with your kids would be better. Your relationship with co-workers would be better. Your relationship with God would be better. In fact, everything about your life would be better. Including your overall health and well-being. Loving others starts with loving self. And loving self starts with squaring your thinking with how God sees you.

The Joy is in the Journey

It's one of my wife's favorite sayings (along with "When are you going to get around to…"). We have conditioned ourselves to believe that joy is in some distant destination we hope to reach some day. I'm not talking about heaven, our ultimate destination. True, the joy of heaven awaits the child of God at the end of life's journey but, even then, I don't think God intends for His children to be miserable along the way. I'm talking about the joy in the journey *now*. Too many people put off being happy and fulfilled because they wait at the end of the dock for their magical ship to come in (of course, they never sent one out). "When I'm able to marry and settle down..." "When I know the joy of little children around my feet..." "When my children leave my feet and go off to college..." "When I'm finally able to retire..." "When we can move to another house..." There's always another carrot to chase. Listen, the joy is in the path we travel *today!* Today matters! It's all you have. Yesterday is gone. Tomorrow is yet to be. You have one day—and it's *today!*

The wise man said, "Indeed, if a man should live many years, let him rejoice in them all" (Ecclesiastes 11:8). Carpe diem! Why would we settle for anything less? Yet most people do. The majority of the population is quite content with mediocrity. They would probably translate Philippians 4:8 to read—

> *Whatever is wrong, whatever is average, whatever is dishonest,*
> *Whatever is impure, whatever is fictitious, whatever is faithless,*
> *Whatever is ugly...negative, worthy of criticism and gossip,*
> *let your mind dwell on these things.*

By the way, all of us are free to choose (and it is a choice!) which version of Philippians 4:8 will guide our thoughts.

It's sad that joyful living is right before our eyes and within our grasp, but we choose not to see it. Julie gets put out with me sometimes because I will go to the pantry in search for the elusive jar of peanut butter and can't find it. So I do what comes natural to the male gender. I say, "Hey, where's the peanut butter?" She says back from the bedroom, "It's on the fourth shelf at eye level." I look and it's not there. It's then I emit male sounds of frustrations. Eventually she stops what she's doing, comes into the kitchen, reaches into the pantry, and hands me the peanut butter. And where was it? On the fourth shelf at eye level—exactly where she said it was. She usually walks away mumbling something about helpless husbands.

The joy of living is right in front of your eyes. If you can't get excited about the love of God, the promises of God, the exceeding joy that Jesus brings to one who has been forgiven and to whom abundant life is offered, I am at a loss as to what other motivation there might be. On the other hand, if you're waiting until everything is perfect in your life before you crack open a smile; you're in for a long wait.

I know what you're thinking… "You have no clue about my struggles with weight…" Okay, I don't. I don't know what you're going through any more than you know what I'm going through (or have gone through). All of us have "issues" and battles we must face and fight. No one is immune. But hear me clearly. Only God can turn a mess into a message. Only God can turn a test into a testimony. Only God can turn a trial into a triumph. And only God can turn a victim into a victory. The question is: Do you trust Him and are you available to Him?

Your Thoughts Are Showing!

I read the other day that the average person has fifty thousand thoughts per day. My immediate thoughts were, how do they know that, and who in their right mind would ever study that? Beats me. Let's just say that the average person has *a lot* of thoughts per day. Those thoughts will either lead you in one or two directions: (1) closer to God, or (2) farther from Him. Don't tell me your thoughts don't matter. They *do* matter and shape who you are each day.

Jesus said, "…for the mouth speaks out of that which fills the heart" (Luke 6:45). The mouth is a tattletale—it tells others what you're thinking. We've all heard someone excuse their caustic comments with, "I'm sorry, I spoke before I thought." Uh, no you didn't. You may not have thought about it long enough (obviously not), but the fact that you spoke it means that you thought it. You cannot divorce your thoughts from your speech and actions. The latter reveals the former.

The problem is…our thoughts tend to be re-treads. Large trucks use re-tread tires on their trailers because they are cheaper. And because they are cheaper, they come apart when the temperature and road surface gets too hot (it's why you have to dodge huge hunks of rubber in the road—known affectionately in trucker-talk as "alligators"). Our thoughts are like that. Because we aren't willing to discipline our minds, we keep rolling out re-tread thoughts. And that's why it's hard to change.

"For as he thinks within himself, so is he" (Proverbs 23:7). And so will he (or she) continue to be as long as the same thoughts are allowed to hang around our mental playground. That's why, if nothing changes (thoughts), nothing changes (behavior). It doesn't matter what kind of change you need to make. It can be physical (weight loss), relationship (making your marriage better), financial (getting your spending under control), spiritual (getting real with God), etc. If you do not fix your thinking, it's going to be a repeat of the same old thing. And...you'll leave a lot of "alligators" in your road for the rest of us to dodge.

Bad Company Sabotages Good Thoughts

Do you know it is impossible to worry without thinking worrisome thoughts? You cannot do it. At the same time, you cannot be afraid without giving in to fearful thoughts. You cannot be depressed without thinking in a direction that makes allowances for that. At the same time, you cannot have hope without thinking hopeful thoughts. You cannot be happy without allowing your mind to be filled with the abundance of God's blessings. You cannot be joyful without thinking thoughts of...*joy*. So, how do I change my thinking?

Here it is: if you hang around negative, faithless, and critical people, guess what you will become? We remind our teens that "bad company corrupts good morals" (1 Corinthians 15:33). Is that applicable only to young people or to *all* people? We fail, however, to note the first part of the verse. It says, "Do not be deceived..." Why did Paul caution about deception before saying that the people in our association will influence us? Because it's easy to be deceived. In fact, we deceive ourselves more than we deceive anyone. We think we can keep company with non-Philippians 4:8 thinkers and it won't matter. But it will matter. Negative people will poison your outlook, exhaust your energy, and steal your joy. And they will tell you again and again that you aren't good enough and/or that any attempt to change will be met with failure. Give them enough of your time and mind and...you will buy into what they're selling.

If you don't believe that, study Numbers 13. When the twelve spies returned from a reconnaissance mission to scope out the Promised Land, ten of the spies returned with a negative report about the fortified cities of Canaan and the size of the giants that lived there. They whined, "We became like grasshoppers in their sight" (v.33). On the other hand, two of the spies (Joshua and Caleb) spoke with glowing confidence in the promises and power of God. *Forget the size of the giants,* they pleaded... *Look at the size of our God!* Now given the two choices (faith or fear), to which did the people adhere? "Then all the congregation lifted up their voices and cried, and the people wept that night. All the sons of Israel grumbled against Moses and Aaron and the whole congregation said to them, 'Would that we had died in the land of Egypt! Or would that we had died in this wilderness!'" (14:1-2). Standing on the shore of the Jordan River, perched to cross over and take God up on His promises, they caved. The pleading of Joshua and Caleb went unheard.

If you associate with those who whine, complain, criticize, or commiserate their troubles, you will fall into the same mental cesspool. "Do not be deceived..." It won't take much to knock you off course.

Sometimes it's our family who nudges us into mediocrity and bad habits. Try as we might, they seem to always be there to pull us back down. This is where the metal of your mental discipline is going to be tested. Can you still believe in yourself when others don't? At some point it will happen. Tell your family that you are embarking on a new journey of health and wholeness and you may get snickers (other than the candy kind). At the end of the day, it may be you and the Lord in your closet of prayer. That's when you're going to need a Joshua or a Caleb. You need a coach, mentor, doctor, trainer—someone to whom you are accountable. Someone who believes in you. Someone who isn't buying your excuses. Someone who will hold you responsible.

And it may cost you. Studies have shown that those who have a financial buy-in with a coach will find greater results. After all, there is truth in the fact that you get what you pay for. Think about the money you spend on junk food and redirect it to someone who can help you. You are, after all, working to regain control of your life. And *you* are worth every penny.

Hit the "OFF" Button

Disaster. Crisis. Failure. Scandal. Danger. Devastation. Terror... were just a few of the words spoken in a five-minute span on a recent newscast. The news channels (all of them) are adept at spreading the gospel of fear and worry. And they do it 24/7/365.

Where your attention goes, your energy flows. Race car legend Mario Andretti was once asked his greatest advice to younger drivers—"Don't look at the wall...Your car goes where your eyes go." It's true. Ask any tightrope walker (I don't know any and you probably don't either—but if you did...), and they will tell you the one thing you must never do is look down. Why? Your body follows your eyes. Your body (your life) follows your eyes (attention). Focus your eyes on constant negative news and your life will reflect the same.

Your mind is like an empty glass. It will retain whatever you put into it. You continue to put in sensational news, salacious headlines, and talk show rants, and you are pouring dirty water into your glass until your thoughts are nothing but a muddy mess. It's the old "garbage in, garbage out." Why would we subject ourselves to those whose job it is to constantly spew dirty water into our glass?

I am not advocating a hermit-type existence that resigns from the real world. It is important to keep up and have a measure of knowledge about the world in which you live. I'm talking about the obsession that some have with the news. I know those who are glued constantly to Fox News and conservative talk radio and who listen to nothing else. It is essential for you to understand that with so much competition on the news front, news producers must stoop to new lows to keep shocking you to pay attention to them and their advertisers (it's all about the money). And they know all too well that nothing grabs your mind faster than a constant dose of old-fashioned fear. In other words, more dirty water.

You only get in life what you expect. And you expect what you think about. So, what drives your thoughts? Answer: whatever you allow yourself to see and hear. And if all you ever feed your mind is the gloom and doom of tragedy, uncertainty, scandals, gossip, and political shenanigans, well, you won't feel very motivated to make any personal changes.

Want good news? You have tremendous power in the palm of your hand. How? Hit the "OFF" button on your remote. Turn off the news. I did. I used to be a news junkie who watched too much cable news and listened to talk radio in the car. No more. It's easy these days to get the headlines in a few seconds to see if anything actually is news worthy (most of the time it is not news reporting but news creating). Then it's on to bigger (and better!) things. Kick the depressing news habit. Improve your outlook by improving your input.

Here is an important fact you must embrace: **control what is controllable.** You can't control the national economy, but you can control your economy. You can't control how the president is running the country, but you can control how you are running your life. You can't control the war in Afghanistan and around the world, but you can control the peace and harmony in your own home. You can't control national healthcare, but you can control the care of your own health. Stop paying attention to what you cannot control, or it will start controlling you.

If you are what you think, then take back your thoughts. Stop letting other people influence your attitude with their sky-is-falling-fear-mongering. Focus your mind on what is right, good, and possible for you. You are surrounded with personal potential every single day. Put your knowledge to work in a positive way and change the world by making a difference in your world. Don't look down, look up!

Basic Training: Boot Camp!

Paul reminds us that we must wear the full armor of God. His description in Ephesians 6:10-17 is that of a Christian soldier. The first thing they do with new soldiers is ship them off to boot camp. 2 Corinthians 10:5 is your boot camp. Here it is: "Take every thought captive to the obedience of Christ." How can you read that verse and conclude that your thoughts don't matter? They do matter. In fact, they are critical to your success or failure (in anything). And he doesn't say, *Take a few thoughts captive and let the others roam free...* No. He says, "Take **every thought** captive to the obedience of Christ." Every thought? Yes, *every thought.* (No one said boot camp was easy).

When our son, Dale, was little he dreamed of being a police officer. He would insist we watch the TV show *Cops* every Saturday night and he knew the words to the "Bad Boy, Bad Boy" song that introduced and closed the program. "When I grow up," he said, "I'm going to be a cop and get the bad guys off the street, handcuff 'em and take 'em to jail!" Guess what? After getting his degree from Western Kentucky University and going on to graduate from the Kentucky police academy at Eastern Kentucky University, he is now a full-fledged law enforcement officer (and has been for several years). I think of him when I think of this verse.

When a non-Philippians 4:8 thought moves into your mental neighborhood and takes up residence, what will you do? You can allow it to set up shop and destroy the good decisions you've already made, or you can throw the handcuffs on that old way of thinking by making the pronouncement— "Not in my neighborhood!" You then march the handcuffed thought before the Judge and if He (Jesus) deems it unworthy, you incarcerate it with a life sentence.

Read it again—"Take every thought captive to the obedience of Christ." Drastic situations require drastic actions. Don't hesitate. By the way, the Magistrate in your mental neighborhood is always available. Never hesitate to approach His bench.

Six Things You Can Do to Guard Your Mind

Remember that you and you alone are the gatekeeper of what you allow into your mind. Blaming your lousy "can't do" attitude on others or your circumstances makes as much sense as blaming the mirror because you don't like the reflection. Take ownership for how you think. Say out loud, "I am responsible for my thoughts, actions, and attitude." Say it again and again until you believe it. You have to believe it because it's true. Okay, let's get down to practical.

1. Clean out the refrigerator. Hopefully you periodically peruse the real one and pitch food with an expired expiration date or throw away the casserole from two weeks ago that now has green mold added to the ingredients. If you don't clean out the'fridge now and then it gets pretty gross.

The same thing is true with your mind. Take inventory as to what is growing in there. "Test yourselves to see if you are in the faith; examine yourselves" (2 Corinthians 13:5). Think about what you're thinking about and figure out *why* you're thinking in that direction. What negative (mold) and self-destructive thoughts (mold) are you allowing to grow in there?

Too much social media? Too much couch-time? Too many excuses? Too many negative people? Clean out the fridge occasionally and if you need to pitch some junk, pitch it.

2. Focus on strong relationships. "Iron sharpens iron, so one man sharpens another" (Proverbs 27:17). Do you associate with those who sharpen your blade or dull it? Invest time with those who see you as God sees you; those who believe in you, those who will hold you accountable and remind you of your successes more than your failures. At the same time, have your antenna up for the joy-thieves. Hang a "No Vacancy" sign at the portal of your mind and determine to let their voices go in one ear and out the other. You don't need that.

3. Meditate upon Scripture. Rather than focusing on an inanimate object on the wall in an attempt to lose your conscious self (the M.O. of Eastern religions), focus instead on Scripture. "Oh how I love Your law, It is my meditation all the day" (Psalm 119:97). I smile when people tell me they can't mediate. I always ask them if they can worry. "Oh yes," is the reply, "I'm very good at that!" Well, if you can worry (negative meditation), you can do the opposite (Philippians 4:8 meditation). Meditating is nothing more than giving serious thought to something. So, give serious thought to that which is true, honorable, right, pure, lovely, excellent, etc. And the best way to do that is to invest thought-time in the Word of God.

4. Personalize Scripture. It's easy to make the Bible so generic that it loses its punch. Insert your name into the verse. For example, "Jesus Christ came that I, _____ (your name) might have life and have it more abundantly" (John 10:10). "In Christ I _____ (your name) live and move and have my being" (Acts 17:28). "I _____ (your name) am transformed by the renewing of my mind" (Rom.12:2). "I _____ (your name) can do all things through Him who strengthens me" (Phil.4:13). Make the promises of God your promises. After all, they are!

5. Quarantine negativity. Simple question: If you're in an elevator and the person next to you starts coughing, sneezing, and hacking, do you try to get closer to that person? Hardly. The same principle applies to negative people. Negative people are contagious. Guard against their viruses. Don't let them get to you.

6. Have an attitude of gratitude. How grateful are you? I don't mean generalized gratitude that we practice daily (as in thanking someone for holding the door). I mean proactive extraordinary gratitude. Gratitude that says I am going to intentionally focus on what is working rather than complain about what isn't. There will always be set-backs and pot-holes. Don't allow them to derail your life. Understand that life on planet Earth is a gift from God and that it is temporary. As a result, treasure the gift of each day and be appreciative of what you have.

Till Your Garden

Galatians 6:7 says, "…for whatever a man sows, this will he also reap." Once more we miss the preamble warning: "Do not be deceived…" Why did he say that again? Because we are prone to deception. Satan has whispered lies since the Garden of Eden, and we continue to believe whatever rolls off his slippery tongue. Stop believing it! If God says you will reap what you sow, then…you will reap…what you sow. Every farmer understands the principle. But it goes beyond that. 2 Corinthians 9:6 adds, "He who sows sparingly will also reap sparingly, and he who sows bountifully will also reap bountifully." While it is true that you will reap what you sow, it is equally true that you will reap *more* than you planted. And every farmer understands that, too.

Our thoughts are like seeds sown into the ground. The life we harvest depends upon the kind of seeds we plant. If you desire a life of joy and satisfaction, then hitch your mind to the joy-producing promises of God. On the other hand, if you allow a few negative, mediocre, and compromising thoughts to take root, you will reap a harvest of bad habits for years to come. Sow a thought, reap a habit. Why? Because thoughts take root. That's why it is essential to till the garden of your mind. Get rid of the weeds or else they will spread. Do not allow anything other than Philippians 4:8 thoughts to grow in your mind.

It's Up to You

When God made you, He gave you a free will. That means He will not force you to eat right, exercise, get your rest, wear your seat belt, read your Bible, pray, be faithful to your spouse, or a hundred other choices you can or cannot make. Right thinking is a choice and it's a choice that He allows you to make. You can live with negative thoughts, be dominated with doubt, and wallow in the drama of uncertainty, or you can make the decision to "renew your mind" and "prove what the will of God is." In other words, you can take charge of your thoughts, seek His counsel, and set a new course as you fulfill His desires for you. As someone said, there are three votes cast. God thinks you can. Satan thinks you can't. The deciding vote is in your hand. So, what do *you* think?

I know, I know. "You can't teach an old dog new tricks." Agreed. But here's some very good news: you are not a dog! You *can* retrain your thoughts. Paul said, "I have *learned* to be content" (Phil.4:11). You can learn.

I don't know who said it, but it's true: **You are the product of your decisions, not your circumstances.** It's easy to blame everyone else and everything else for the mess you're in. And as long as you keep doing that, nothing will change. Take ownership. While you can't always choose your circumstances, you can always choose your attitude and response. Keep in mind the attitude you choose is a direct reflection of your faith in God.

Basketball coaches sometime sense the game is getting away from their team and will call a well-placed "time out!" The coach calls the team to his side, looks each player in the eye and says, "Get your head in the game!" Why does he challenge them with such severity? Because he sees their minds have wandered, and they are not focused. Sometimes *our* minds wander, too. The problem is; this is not a game. This is life. This is *your* life. And this is the *only life* you have. Refocus. Recommit. Reengage.

The secret to anything is a commitment to the NOW. You must square your thinking *today*. The person who says, "I'll start working on my marriage, finances, spiritual life, or health *tomorrow...*" has already failed. God gives to each of us the invaluable gift of right now. It is the present of the *present*. What are you going to do with it?

Philippians 4:8 will change your life. But...it's up to *you*.

Epilogue

*So choose life in order that you may live…by loving the Lord your God,
by obeying His voice, and by holding fast to Him; for this is your life
and the length of your days.* (Deuteronomy 30:19-20)

I write this while more than halfway through my fifty-fifth year. I have dedicated this year to finding my halftime (some may think I'm a little late for that). Let's just say it's like the Super Bowl—after all, they have a long halftime. Like every basketball or football game, a team plays the first half to get to the second half. It's during halftime that coaches and players take stock, make adjustments, reassess, and tweak the game plan. The first half is a lot of hype and hoopla. Even before the game begins they turn out the arena lights, shine the spotlights, and play loud "Are—You—Ready—For—This" music. Kind of like when you were born. You hadn't as yet accomplished anything (except show up), yet family and friends are yelling and screaming your name (okay, *quiet* yelling and screaming) while taking hundreds of pictures. Welcome to the Opening Ceremonies.

My son Luke and I attended a University of Louisville versus Syracuse basketball game in January of this year at the Yum Center in Louisville. That's "Yum" as in the Yum Corporation—owners of Taco Bell, Pizza Hut, and Kentucky Fried Chicken (the world's largest fast food company in terms of units—39,000 restaurants around the world). Irony aside, even though the University of Louisville went on to win the NCAA national championship in men's basketball later in the year, they blew that game—*in the second half.* By the way, the game is usually won or lost in the second half. You can make mistakes in the first half and still have time to recover.

That's where halftime happens. The second half, however, is crunch time. The second half is where everything is on the line. Game on.

Bob Buford's book, *Halftime—Moving from Success to Significance* is one of the best books I've ever read. He captures the essence of where so many of us baby-boomers are (and everyone else eventually will be). He writes, "During the first half of your life, if you are like me, you probably did not have time to think about how you would spend the rest of your life. You probably rushed through college, fell in love, married, embarked on a career, climbed upward, and acquired a few things to help make the journey comfortable. You played a hard-fought first half. You even may be winning. But sooner or later you begin to wonder if this really is as good as it gets." Been there, thought that. I doubt I'm the only one.

Here's the deal. America in the twenty-first century needs an entirely new paradigm shift when it comes to life. The old (go to college, get a job, work until you're sixty, retire, and rock on the porch at Cracker Barrel) is old school. Listen, given life expectancy these days, we have a lot of life left. But only if… you take care of yourself. And you can't wait until you are sixty to start.

If I may tweak Bob Buford's concept of *Halftime—From Success to Significance*, here is what I would say.

First Half		Second Half
Who am I?		Discovering a purpose beyond self
What do I believe?		What I do about what I believe
Faith means giving up things	**HALFTIME**	Faith means addition and abundance
Me versus them ("What's in it for me?")		Us
Sowing, planting, and earning		Harvesting, listening, and learning
Based on externals/appearances		Based on internals ("As a man thinks…")
Authoritarian leadership		Servant leader
Success-driven		Significance-driven
A Sunday focused Christian		A seven-day-a-week-focused Christian
Health concerns—*Tomorrow…*		Health concerns—*Today!*

Do you see a difference? Obviously this represents some overlapping and oversimplification. For example, I hope you figured out some of the second half stuff *before* halftime. By and large, however, the second half is when knowledge transforms into wisdom.

Someone said that a successful first thirty, forty, fifty years should only be considered a good start. The question is; what are you going to do now? How are you going to live? What decisions will you make that will enable the best years of your life to be the ones still to come?

Maybe you need to stop, take inventory, and reassess. I hope something in this book has motivated you to do exactly that. Maybe you need to find your halftime; your turning point.

The Best Is Yet to Be

This has been the best year of my life. I have more energy. I feel better. I go to bed earlier. I get up at dawn. I enjoy my early morning coffee and quiet time. I quit watching the depressing (and time-wasting) news. I read voraciously. I write every day. I don't work with the largest church around, but it's one of the best. I teach and tell people about Jesus. I'm madly in love with my wife. I've learned and am still learning what a God-send treasure she is. I'm also learning a lot about real love—which means I'm also learning a lot about God since "God is love." And I'm trying to take much better care of myself.

I've learned to say "No, thank you..." when sharing a meal in someone's home when they have a tempting dessert. Okay, if it's too tempting, I've learned to eat a smaller portion. I haven't had a drink all year (that sounds funny) except water. I added up all those extra liquid calories and guess what I found? ZERO PLUS ZERO = ZERO! Occasionally I'll get a *hankering* (I'm from Tennessee, remember) for a soft drink, but I'll just refill my lemon-lime water that Julie keeps in the fridge. We don't even buy soft drinks any more. We eat more chicken and fish and less of the fried fare. Fast food restaurants are for "emergencies only" (most have grilled chicken salads).

We exercise. I would like to say we work out every day without exception. Sunday, however, is our exception. It's a day we focus on higher things. Sure, other things can get in the way on other days, too. And that's okay. No worries and no stress. We've decided not to make this life change a big deal. Simple changes over time add up to positive benefits. By the way, making no changes adds up, too.

Our one vice is coffee. We love our coffee. In fact, we love coffee so much that for a time we owned a coffee shop near Nashville (until two ladies came in one day, fell in love with the place, and bought it...but that's another story all together). Our Keurig machine works overtime. However, we drink ours black. No cream. No sugar. Just coffee—the way it was meant to be. The way I used to drink it as a kid sitting at the kitchen table with my grandmother listing to the local morning radio show in Fulton, Kentucky ("The Live Wire") where they did live remotes to the funeral home, hospital, and police station announcing all the goings-on from the previous night. I think that was before they had any HIPPA laws).

My favorite time of the day is sunrise. It is so tranquil and peaceful. It brings calm. It's a time for reflection, thinking, reading, and praying. Mark 1:35 gives us a peek into Jesus' routine. "In the early morning, while it was still dark, Jesus got up, left the house, and went away to a secluded place and was praying there." That speaks to me.

My early morning routine is a big part of my turning point. Nothing begins the day better than to see the sun burst forth across a fog-shrouded Tennessee field with a cup of coffee in one hand and a book in the other. It brings focus. It brings clarity. It reminds me that life is good; that God is good.

I have no idea where you are in life or what life experiences you have faced. But I would hope that you would do everything possible to stay in as good a shape as you can to be of service to the Creator and for those He has placed in your path. The decisions you make today about your health and well-being may determine how active and available you will be in a few short years. Your health will catch up with you and quickly. What then?

Last Saturday Julie and I took our five-year-old grandson Gavin on a five-hour canoe trip. It was fantastic. She paddled, I paddled, and Gavin tried to paddle. He mostly kept his oar in the water reaching to scoop up leaves or whatever else he could find (it was similar to driving with the emergency brake partially on). Regardless, we made a memory. I am thankful I have the health to make those memories. I plan on making many, many more.

Tarzan and Jane Sittin' in a Tree...

Eat right and exercise. Eat right and exercise. Blah. Blah. Blah. We know the *what*. Information isn't the problem with most of us. Sadly, and I hate to say this, but...when it comes to this subject—especially when it comes to *this subject*—we don't like to be told what to do. That's it! For some odd reason we *hate* doing what we know we should be doing. So, we decide to solve the problem by despising the messenger—any messenger—who would dare tell us what we already know we should be doing. It's the old, "Nobody is going to tell me what to do."

So, don't do it.

Seriously, don't do it. No one is forcing you to do anything. I'll state it plainly: You do not have to get in shape. I'll even underline it: <u>You do not have to get in shape.</u> You can do with your body whatever you wish. It's up to you. But I will promise you something...the years will come and go (faster than you wish), and the decisions you make about your health will eventually work for you or against you. Sure, we were born to die. I've got that. But wouldn't you rather enjoy a life well-managed until God calls you home than merely existing from day to day wishing He would? Walk the halls of the nursing or assisted living home. Few of those folks seem to be enjoying their remaining years. Is that how you want to end?

Staying in good shape isn't nearly as complex and daunting as our media-drenched culture pretends it to be. I mean, come on. How hard is it to walk a mile or two every day? How hard is it to drink water instead of a sugar soda? How hard is it to buy some fruit and eat it? Habits form from what we do daily. Get used to drinking water, and you'll choose it again. Get used to exercising, and you'll find out you like it. Eating right and working out isn't about trying to get ripped like Tarzan so you can swing from tree to tree and impress Jane. It's about taking care of you so you can be there for Jane and for all those grandkids. After all, someone has to be around to show them the ropes (or vines).

Where Do We Go from Here?

People want simplistic solutions to complex problems. Usually they want the government to fix it. That isn't going to happen. After fifty-five plus years, here's what I've discovered. I cannot fix the world. I cannot fix Washington or Wall Street. I cannot fix my state, my county, my city, or even my little subdivision. But I can work hard to fix me.

We are facing the perfect storm of processed foods, fast foods, and societal sedentary habits that has helped to shape us (and that "shape" isn't very good). The same storm will cripple the next generation and the health care system as we know it. Sure, we can have more government regulations, educational programs, stricter advertising guidelines, specific warnings labels on foods, more greenways, bike paths, gym classes, and dozens of other plans and programs, but at the end of the day it all comes down to you and me and the daily choices we make for ourselves and our families. As Dr. David Katz said in Mika Brzezinski's *Obsessed*, "We would not countenance building a house out of junk. We would not sanction driving a car built out of junk. And yet we look every day at children being built out of junk and everybody's okay with it. There's something profoundly wrong with that." He's right.

Oddly enough, while poverty in third world countries invites starvation, in the U.S. it invites obesity. It's just easier (and cheaper) to eat calorie dense yet nutrient deficient junk food and feed a constant diet of the same to our kids. As a result, our kids succumb to what used to be adult-onset diabetes, a rising rate of stroke, and shorter life expectancies. If you doubt that, you simply have not been paying attention. Look around. Sure, starvation can kill a child. But so can other chronic diseases that come on slowly and rob years from their life or rob life from their years.

Have we reached the point where it's okay to cheat our children from health and wellness just because the consequences come on gradually? If so, who could argue against letting our kids smoke cigarettes? After all, it wouldn't kill them...*immediately.*

Family is the basic unit of society and in that unity we find our strength. Together we can stand and make healthy lifestyle changes. It comes down to you and me. Someone has to be the responsible adult in the room, set a better example and develop better habits. You can take a look around and figure out that, as a whole, we haven't done a very good job. Obviously you can't stop your kids from eating junk when they are out of your sight, but you can give them the information and the example they need to make better overall choices. Kids do model their parents. Like father, like son. Like mother, like daughter.

You have to take charge of your life. You have to take charge of your family's life. No blame. No excuses. The buck stops here, and the buck stops now.

I know, I know. It sometimes feels overwhelming and like you're up against the tide. Consider this...

A little girl was seen on the shore throwing starfish back into the ocean swells. A storm had swept in washing thousands ashore and leaving them helpless and soon to die from the rising sun. The small child took it upon herself to save one after another. An old man happened along. Cynical and disapproving, he scowled, "My child, you cannot possibly make a difference to all these starfish—seeing there are thousands upon thousands of them." To that discouragement she merely knelt down, picked up another starfish, and threw it back into the water. She then looked at the old man and said, "I made a difference to that one!" The old man smiled. He then gently knelt beside her and together they threw back as many as they could.

"I made a difference to that one..." That "one" starts with me. And it starts now. Care to join the journey?

Thanks for staying, sharing your time, and listening.
I would love to hear from you.
You may contact me via Facebook.

3C Wellness Academy

Carter Hays combines faith, fitness, and performance to deliver more than 35+ years as a recognized expert in the field of fitness. Offering effective exercise, nutrition, and lifestyle strategies, his clients include contestants from the NBC TV show, *The Biggest Loser*, athletes from all the major sports, and people in everyday walks of life.

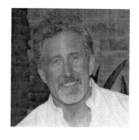

Working in the Nashville, Tennessee area, Carter offers both personal training and group instruction. Twice each year, he hosts "Unleash The Champion"—a weeklong event (spring) and weekend event (fall) at a retreat tucked away at a beautiful lodge in the Tennessee countryside. With guest speakers including former *Biggest Loser* contestants, doctors, authors, nutritionists, etc., its purpose is to educate the mind as well as provide walks and workouts that encourage the CAN DO spirit in anyone regardless of shape and size.

It may be the one vacation you will talk about for the rest of your life.

Contact him via Facebook or visit his website at **www.3cwellnessacademy.com** for more information.

Juice PLUS⁺ The Next Best Thing to Fruits and Vegetables

Juice Plus+ is whole food based nutrition, including juice powder concentrate from 25 different fruits, vegetables, and grains. Everyone wants to eat right and maintain a healthier lifestyle—whether you're a busy mom hustling to feed on-the-go children, a business traveler trying to stay fit, or an active baby-boomer keeping up with grandkids.

All of us try to eat better for good health, but a healthy diet is often a challenge. We simply don't eat enough fruits and vegetables. And that hurts our health and wellness. Juice Plus+ bridges the gap between what you should eat and what you do eat every day.

Not a multivitamin, medicine, treatment or cure for any disease, Juice Plus+ is all-natural and made from quality ingredients carefully monitored from farm to capsule (or gummy) so you can enjoy improved nutrition and wellness.

For more information, visit **www.julieadamsjuiceplus.com**.

Other Books by Wilson Adams

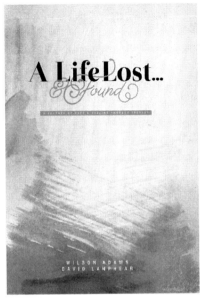

When life takes an uncertain turn, friends Wilson Adams and David Lanphear are unafraid. They have already journeyed through heartbreaking losses to find healing and hope—and they want the same for you.

Packed with Scripture and insight, *A Life Lost...and Found* offers help to those who have walked through the valley of the shadows of suffering. Whether impacted by death, divorce, or disease, this book will take you from the shadows of despair to blue skies and rainbows of hope.

The authors are also available for speaking engagements on the subject of grief. Contact Wilson Adams via Facebook.

Both *Around the House* and *Around the House...Again!* are collections of stories dealing with common life experiences. Sometimes serious, sometimes lighthearted; they will always make you think. And... appreciate the blessings of life.

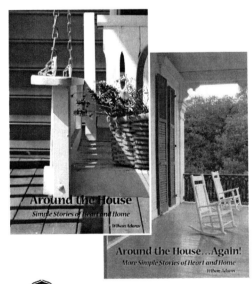

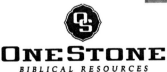

ONE STONE
BIBLICAL RESOURCES

Order from www.OneStone.com

Courageous Living Series
by Wilson Adams

24 Titles Currently Available

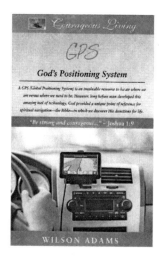

The Courageous Living Bible Study Series has been developed to aid in adult Bible studies. It is designed for everything from one-on-one studies to large group adult Bible classes.

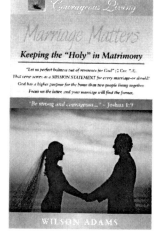

This series of study guides will fit well with any church's adult curriculum. Additionally, some churches have used them effectively in college classes.

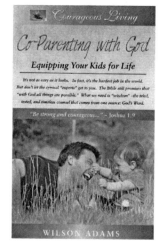

Each approximately 60-page workbook follows the same format: four pages of easy-to-read, fully outlined texts, followed by one page called "Digging Deeper" (thought and discussion-style questions). There are twelve lessons per book. Currently, there are 24 titles in this series, and as new workbooks are added, they can be viewed at www.onestone.com.

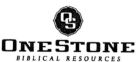

ONE STONE
BIBLICAL RESOURCES

Order from www.OneStone.com

CPSIA information can be obtained at www.ICGtesting.com
Printed in the USA
LVOW10s0331081214

417724LV00021B/321/P

9 780985 493899